Low Fat, Low Sugar

Rose Elliot is Britain's foremost vegetarian cookery writer and her books have won her popular acclaim in all parts of the English-speaking world.

Rose has been in the vanguard of the revolution in our eating habits in recent years, as more and more people consume less meat and take greater interest in healthy eating. She frequently contributes to magazines, gives cookery demonstrations and broadcasts on radio and television. Rose is also a professional astrologer and, with her husband, runs a computer-based astrological service which provides personality profiles, forecasts and compatibility charts. (For more details, please send SAE to Rose Elliot, PO Box 16, Eastleigh SO5 6BH, UK.)

D0348774

Other books by Rose Elliot

Vegan Feasts
Cheap and Easy
The Bean Book

Low Fat, Low Sugar

ROSE ELLIOT

Thorsons

Thorsons
An Imprint of HarperCollins*Publishers*
77-85 Fulham Palace Road,
Hammersmith, London W6 8JB

The Thorsons website address is: www.thorsons.com

Published by Thorsons 2000

10 9 8 7 6 5 4 3

Copyright © Rose Elliot 2000

Rose Elliot asserts the moral right to
be identified as the author of this work

Text illustrations by Helen Holroyd

A catalogue record for this book
is available from the British Library

ISBN 0 7225 3949 5

Printed and bound in Great Britain by
Martins the Printers Limited,
Berwick upon Tweed

All rights reserved. No part of this publication may be
reproduced, stored in a retrieval system, or transmitted,
in any form, or by any means, electronic, mechanical,
photocopying, recording or otherwise, without the prior
permission of the publishers.

This book is sold subject to the condition that it shall not,
by way of trade or otherwise, be lent, re-sold, hired out or
otherwise circulated without the publisher's prior consent
in any form of binding or cover other than that in which it
is published and without a similar condition including this
condition being imposed on the subsequent purchaser.

contents

introduction

When my publisher suggested the idea of Low Fat, Low Sugar, the aim was to write a book which would be helpful to two groups of people: those who, for reasons of health, had to cut down on the amount of fat they were eating, and those who, for the same reason, had to reduce their sugar intake. It was not until I began work on the book and started researching the subject that I began to understand how closely these two issues – our consumption of fat and sugar – are linked in the overall picture of a healthy diet. And as I studied the facts I realised that a diet low in fat and sugar is not only the way to ease – and perhaps even cure – certain diseases but it can also help prevent them occurring in the first place. In addition, following such a diet is a simple and effective way to feel positively healthy and full of energy whilst controlling your weight – even losing some if you need to. I hope therefore that this book will be useful to you, whether you have to change your diet for health reasons or want to make a positive life style change for a slimmer, healthier, happier you.

SO, WHY LOW FAT, LOW SUGAR?

The advantages of a low-fat diet – for slimming, reducing cholesterol, treating heart problems and arteriosclerosis, diabetes and gall bladder problems – are well known and widely advocated. There are many low-fat foods in the supermarkets and low-fat cookbooks in the bookshops. Few, if any of these, however, address the other very important issue: sugar. In fact, manufacturers of low-fat foods frequently enhance the flavour of their products with extra sugar in an effort to make them taste good. It is therefore difficult to find convenience foods that are both low fat and low sugar. Yet, as you will discover, sugar and fat are intricately linked. It doesn't make much sense to cut down on the fats only to stoke up with the sugars. I believe that a truly healthy diet is not only low in fat but low in sugar too.

SUGAR SENSE

We used to think that the main problem with eating sugar was that it rotted our teeth. In fact what happens after the sugar has left our mouth is much more serious and damaging. Sugar stimulates our pancreas to secrete insulin, one of the body's most powerful hormones, in order to regulate the amount of sugar getting into our bloodstream. The insulin deals with the sugar by getting the body to store it as fat; and at the same time the liver produces more cholesterol. Insulin also makes it harder for the body to get rid of stored fat.

Refined carbohydrates such as bread and biscuits also produce sugar in the blood are dealt with by the body in the same way as sugar. Although wholegrain cereals such as real wholemeal (wholewheat) bread are also digested in the same way, the process is slower and the quantity of insulin needed is smaller. This is because the bran and natural fibre they contain prevents them from being broken down and absorbed too quickly: nature has provided an in-built brake. Such foods are therefore excellent sources of slow-release energy, in addition to the many vitamins and minerals they contain.

It is now thought that one of the reasons for the large increase in mature-onset diabetes in developed countries is the increased consumption of sugar and refined carbohydrates that has come about through mass production. Eating these foods regularly strains the body's delicate mechanism for dealing with them until eventually it is unable to operate properly. It is clear that a healthy diet has to be low in sugar and in refined carbohydrates.

FAT FACTS

There are three main types of fat, each classified according to its chemical structure: saturated fat, polyunsaturated fat and monounsaturated fat. They do not all affect the body in the same way (except for piling on the pounds if we eat too much of them – unfortunately they all have this in common).

Saturated fats are found mainly in animal fats – meat, butter, lard, milk and eggs. Fish contains 10–25 per cent. There is little saturated fat in plant oils, with the exception of palm oil and coconut oil which are often included in soft margarines. Saturated fats raise the levels of cholesterol in the blood. This can lead to heart disease and some types of cancer and the general recommendation is that we should reduce our intake of these fats as much as possible.

Polyunsaturated fats are found in greatest quantities in plants, particularly soya, corn, cottonseed, wheatgerm, sunflower and safflower. Most animal products contain very little, although fish is rich in omega-3 fatty acids which are a type of polyunsaturated fat.

Monounsaturated fats are found in many foods including nuts, butter, meat, eggs, milk and margarines, but the most concentrated source is olive oil, which contains 70–90 per cent. Rape seed oil and avocados are also rich in monounsaturated fats. Neither polyunsaturated nor monounsaturated fats raise the level of cholesterol in the blood and when included in the diet both reduce the risk of heart disease.

SO WHY BOTHER TO CUT BACK ON THESE FATS?

Our intake of fat affects the amount of cholesterol in our bloodstream and our vulnerability to diseases affecting the heart and arteries, as well as our suseptibility to gallstones. Fats of any kind have more than double the number of calories per gram than either of the other main food groups – proteins and sugars. In addition, calories from fat are more easily stored as fat in our bodies than calories from other sources. So a diet high in fat increases the risk of obesity, and both obesity and a diet high in fat may increase the risk of certain cancers.

In America and Britain we obtain, on average, almost 40 per cent of our calories from fat. This percentage is beginning to fall because of the availability of low-fat foods and our awareness of their value to our health. However, we have quite a way to go, because a healthy percentage is considered to be 15–30 per cent. In fact in a traditional Asian diet, with its low incidence of heart disease, diabetes and cancer, fat supplies only 15–22 per cent of calories.

There are some doctors who consider even 15–22 per cent too high. The late Dr Nathan Pritikin, founder of the Pritikin Longevity Centers in California, set the target at 10 per cent. His methods have helped tens of thousands of people lose weight and keep it off, as well as helping reduce or eliminate medication for heart and arterial problems, high blood pressure and diabetes, and in some cases reversing the patient's disease. Similar results are reported by Dr Dean Ornish, who also advocates a diet containing not more than 10 per cent fat and one that is based entirely on pulses, fruits, grains, vegetables and small quantities of fat-free dairy products. The results of these pioneering doctors are inspiring because they show how the body can heal itself, given the right diet and exercise.

HOW LOW CAN YOU GO?

A completely fat-free diet would be unhealthy. Our bodies need to take in 4–6 per cent of calories as fat in order to be able to synthesise the essential fatty acids necessary for health. If you kept strictly to the Pritikin diet, Dr Dean Ornish's diet or indeed the recipes given in this book, you would be getting about 10 per cent of your calories from fat; this being derived from the small amounts naturally present in whole grains, pulses, fruits, vegetables and low-fat dairy produce. The good news is that although these ingredients are low in fat, they contribute the vital nutrients which your body needs to heal itself and to function at its peak.

There are some practitioners who advocate supplementing our general diet with Essential Fatty Acids (EFA's) either in the form of oil or capsules. A diet which is very low in fat allows you the leeway to include these valuable oils if you wish. They could be particularly beneficial to vegetarians, who are not getting any of the omega-oils from fish. Look for 'Udo's oils' in health food stores, or ask the staff for advice. These oils need to be kept in the refrigerator and used up quickly.

CURING CANDIDIASIS

The recipes in this book are, like those of Dr Pritikin and Dr Ornish, based on the ingredients mentioned above. However, because I wanted this book to be useful for those suffering from yeast-related problems – the effects of an overgrowth of Candida albicans (candiasis) – I have also excluded other ingredients. There are no fruits or artificial sweeteners in the recipes; also excluded are yeast and products containing it; vinegar and fermented products, including soy sauce; malted products; anything containing mould, such as cheese; and mushrooms. Milk and most products made from it are also unsuitable because they contain lactic acid, which is a form of sugar. The exception is yogurt, which is allowed because most of the lactose has been digested by the bacteria present in the yogurt. So low-fat yogurt is suitable, even though other milk products are not.

Stimulants – tea, coffee, chocolate and cola drinks – also have to go because they cause the adrenal glands to trigger the release of the body's sugar stores into the bloodstream, 'feeding' the candida in the same way as sugar in the digestive system. Caffeine is also banned from the Pritikin program, and by Dr Ornish. If you go to a nutritional therapist the first thing they will do, most likely, is tell you to give up coffee (and some will ban tea, too). Although it's the caffeine which is the main problem, many practitioners recommend you avoid both normal and de-caffeinated coffee.

Having loved both tea and coffee, particularly the latter, dark and strong as could be, I could never imagine myself not drinking them. However, I have now given them up and I would not have believed how much better I feel. I mainly drink rooibosh tea, made from the seed of the redbush tree, in place of both tea and coffee. It has a flavour not unlike tea and although it took me a while to like it as much as I used to like tea, I can now say that I do. (But not as much as real coffee. My body likes it a lot better, though.) If you do come off tea and coffee, be prepared for some withdrawal symptoms – probably headaches – in the first few days. Take painkillers for these if you need to, but make sure that these do not contain caffeine.

If you suspect that you may be suffering from candida, symptoms of which range from chronic fatigue to aching joints and muscles and a weakened immune system, you can cure yourself by keeping to a strict diet and taking vitamin and anti-fungal supplements. I recommend Erica White's *Beat Candida Cookbook* published by Thorsons for more information on this subject.

a personal note

When I write a cookery book I generally put on a pound or two in weight – an inevitable side-effect of all the tasting and testing which has to be done. It's irritating, and a nuisance having to lose the weight afterwards; in fact it's the one aspect of recipe writing that I don't enjoy. During the writing of this book, however, it was different. When I'd finished I found that not only had I not gained the usual weight but I'd actually lost over half a stone without thinking about it or trying. The food was delicious and I had lots of energy. I hope it's the same for you.

low-fat, low-sugar ingredients

After all my comments about foods which are not used in this book you're probably wondering what on earth you can eat. Actually it's surprising how many ingredients are suitable:

Fresh vegetables: all kinds can be eaten – raw or cooked, in soups, salads, main courses and, in the case of some of the sweeter ones such as butternut squash, as the basis for desserts and cakes. Choose organic if possible to avoid the risk of chemical residues. If you can't manage to go completely organic, do choose organic carrots, lettuces and soya (also bananas, strawberries, milk and chocolate if you're eating these). I'd also like to add organic potatoes to that list and hope that it won't be very long before organic produce is the norm rather than the exception in all our food shops.

Frozen and canned vegetables: some of these are useful but make sure that they do not contain added sugar. Look for organic tomatoes canned without citric acid, particularly if you're on the diet to combat candida. Canned sweetcorn without added sugar or salt is useful; also frozen sweetcorn, peas and broad beans.

Lemons: the only fruit permitted, apart from a little lime rind and juice which I've used very occasionally. Lemon juice is used instead of vinegar in dressings and a squeeze at the end of cooking is a useful flavour-enhancer in many dishes. Buy unwaxed, preferably organic lemons, especially if you're going to use the skins as well as the juice.

Pulses: dried beans and lentils are wonderful, virtually fat-free sources of protein, fibre, minerals and vitamins. Many recipes in this book include these in either their dried or canned form. Again, buy organic if you can. Canned organic pulses are now available from large supermarkets and health food stores and are very handy, though dried pulses are easy to prepare.

To prepare pulses, cover with cold water and soak for 8 hours, or bring to the boil and leave to soak for 1 hour. Rinse and cover generously with fresh cold water. Boil rapidly for 10 minutes before reducing the heat and letting them boil gently until tender: usually

1–1½ hours. Lentils and split peas cook in 20–60 minutes, depending on the type – they don't need soaking before cooking although if you do soak them they cook more quickly. All pulses freeze well. For convenience, cook a 500g/18oz bag, divide into 5 portions and freeze – each portion will be the equivalent of a 425g/15oz can of beans.

Whole grains: this group includes brown rice, quinoa, millet and flaked brown rice, as well as brown rice flour and polenta (maize flour). Couscous is a refined, not a whole grain; bulgur wheat is a more nutritious alternative and is just as easy to prepare. Wholewheat pasta is also very useful in the diet. If you can't eat wheat, non-wheat pastas made from vegetables, corn, millet and rice are available from health food stores.

Tofu: this useful and nutritious ingredient is used in quite a few of the recipes. It's particularly important to buy an organic type to ensure that it hasn't been made from GM soya beans.

Low-fat plain organic yogurt: If you can't tolerate any dairy produce, use an unsweetened soya yogurt instead. You can buy this from health food stores, or it's easy to make your own (see page 151).

Soya milk: unsweetened organic soya milk is used in recipes instead of dairy milk.

Organic free-range eggs: egg whites are used in a few of the recipes in this book.

Cold-pressed organic olive oil: this is used only in a handful of the recipes. If you wish to add a light misting of oil to vegetables before roasting or frying, you might like to make an oil spray by putting some olive oil into a spray bottle, topping up with 8 parts of cold water and shaking and spraying when required.

Spices: apart from the very hot spices, such as chilli and cayenne, these are usually allowed and are invaluable for making low-fat, low-sugar meals taste really good. A particular favourite in this book is cumin, in both seed and powdered form; ground coriander and turmeric are also invaluable, as is nutmeg – buy it whole and grate as required. Freshly ground black pepper can also be used freely. Buy the spices as you need them for a particular recipe and you'll soon build up a useful collection.

Fresh herbs: I think the availability of a wide range of fresh herbs is one of the factors that has made the most impact on our cooking in the last ten years. They are a wonderful way of adding freshness and flavour to dishes and make a very appetising garnish. Fresh ginger and garlic are also indispensable flavourings.

Salt: may not be recommended by most health experts, but it is difficult to reduce while still retaining flavour. As a substitute, I have recently been using a sodium-reduced sea salt from Iceland. It is the best of the reduced sodium salts that I have tried. Reduced sodium salts contain a higher percentage of potassium than normal salt, so if you're having treatment for a kidney or heart disorder, check with your doctor before using it.

equipment and techniques

The only special equipment needed for low-fat, low-sugar cooking is one or two non-stick pans: ideally, a large non-stick frying pan with a lid and a medium-sized saucepan for making sauces and other mixtures that tend to stick. A non-stick baking sheet or tray is also useful or, alternatively, you could buy some of the non-stick fabric which you simply place on an ordinary baking tray. It can be washed and re-used time and again.

DRY-FRYING

The recipes in this book are fairly simple and do not involve complicated techniques. However, what I call 'dry-frying' is used in quite a number of the dishes. This is simply cooking in a frying pan or saucepan (non-stick) without added oil or liquid. By dry-frying an onion, for instance, you can get a result very much like fried onion. Put a fairly finely chopped onion into the frying pan, cover with a lid and set over a gentle heat. Let it cook for 6–7 minutes, stirring often. It will soften and become lightly flecked with brown. Turn up the heat if you want to brown it more, but take care because it's easy to burn it and get a bitter flavour. If this seems likely, add a little water or stock and continue to gently 'fry' the onion until the liquid has disappeared and the onion is tender.

You can use this technique with any vegetable if you want a fried effect without using fat. If using no fat seems too extreme, you could try using just a teaspoonful of olive oil. It's surprising how little you need. When I started experimenting with recipes for this book I initially used a teaspoonful of oil for the frying process, but having tried frying onions without any oil, decided to opt for this 'purer' approach which seemed to give results which were just as good. Once you start using little bits of oil here and little bits there, it starts to add up and the diet stops being 'low fat'. However, how low you go is up to you; because the recipes are strict you have the scope to add a little fat here and there where it matters to you. One tablespoonful of oil adds 15 grams of fat to a recipe; a teaspoonful adds 5 grams of fat.

THE OIL AND WATER SPRAY

I think the idea for this originally came from low-fat cook extraordinaire Sue Kreitz-man. All you do is buy a small spray bottle at a chemist or garden centre, fill this with olive oil and water in the proportion of 1 part oil to 8 or 10 parts water, shake well, then spray over your food. I use this on Mediterranean vegetables such as aubergines (eggplants) and courgettes (zucchini), or on burgers and rissoles before grilling or baking them. An alternative would be to use one of the oil sprays which you can buy in supermarkets, but making your own is so easy and you know exactly what's in it. The only time when a supermarket oil spray is useful is for greasing cake tins (pans), although if you use non-stick baking parchment you don't need it.

When making a soup I generally start by sautéing an onion and any other vegetables in a tablespoonful of olive oil or a small amount of butter, as I have found that this gives the soup a superior flavour. However, wanting to keep the recipes as 'pure' as possible, I also experimented with dry-frying the onion and other vegetables before adding the stock or water and found that this also worked well. This process seems to draw out the flavour and, if you allow the vegetables to brown, caramelises their natural sugars and adds to the finished taste of the soup. So after much testing and experimenting, I decided to use this method as a basis for many of the soups. However, if you want to add a little fat, sautéing in 1 teaspoon of olive oil will usually add only about 1 gram of fat per serving.

Good stock can also contribute enormously to the success of a soup and is not difficult to come by now that you can buy vegetable stock in supermarkets or make up your own from good quality stock cubes or – my favourite – vegetable bouillon powder.

Of course in low-fat cookery you can't rely on a splash of cream to add the final touch to soup and a spoonful of low-fat yogurt somehow doesn't have the same effect. I think that often the nicest finishing touch is a generous scattering of chopped fresh herbs, which are easy to get almost anywhere all the year round.

flageolet bean, leek and watercress soup

Pale green flageolet beans give this soup a delicate flavour, plentiful nutrients and a slightly thickened texture. You can buy them in cans at large supermarkets.

serves 4

2 leeks, sliced
425g/15oz can flageolet beans
600ml/20fl oz/2½ cups vegetable stock or water
1 bunch or packet of watercress
salt and freshly ground black pepper

Put the leek into a non-stick pan, cover and cook very gently for about 7 minutes, until the leek is becoming tender, stirring from time to time. Drain and rinse the beans, then add them to the pan along with the stock or water. Bring to the boil, then reduce the heat, cover and leave to boil gently for 10–15 minutes, stirring occasionally, until the leeks are fully cooked. Put a ladleful of the soup into a food processor or blender with the watercress and whiz to a purée. Return this to the saucepan, stir and season with salt and freshly ground black pepper. Bring back to just below boiling point and serve.

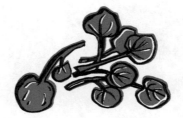

roasted butternut squash soup with cumin

Butternut squash has a glorious dense golden flesh with a very sweet flavour. I think the best way to cook it, to bring out all the flavour, is to bake it. The squash can be baked in advance, when convenient, then you can whiz up this delicious soup in the minimum of time.

serves 4

Preheat the oven to 200°C/400°F/gas mark 6.

Cut the squash in half, down through its stem. Scoop out the seeds, then put the halves cut-side down on to a baking tray and bake for 45–60 minutes, or until they are tender, turning them over about half way through cooking time. Cool. Scoop the flesh away from the skin using a spoon and discard the skin. All this can be done well in advance if convenient.

When you're ready to make the soup, put the onion into a non-stick pan, cover and cook gently for about 7 minutes, until the onion is tender and lightly browned, stirring from time to time. Add the garlic and cumin, stir over the heat for a few seconds, until the cumin smells aromatic, then add the squash flesh and the stock or water. Bring to the boil, reduce the heat and leave to boil gently for about 10 minutes, to allow all the flavours to blend and to ensure everything is cooked. Purée in a food processor or blender. Add a little more stock or water if necessary to get the consistency to your liking. Season with salt and freshly ground black pepper and serve.

1 butternut squash
1 onion, chopped
1 large garlic clove, chopped
1tsp ground cumin
600ml/20fl oz/2½ cups vegetable stock or water
salt and freshly ground black pepper

lentil and carrot soup

Lentil soup is always soothing and sustaining, and this is a particularly delicious recipe for this favourite. If you have a pressure cooker, you can speed up the cooking time by cooking at high pressure, after the lentils and stock or water have been added, for 5 minutes.

serves 4

2 onions, chopped
2 carrots, sliced
225g/8oz/heaping 1 cup red lentils
1 litre/35fl oz/4½ cups vegetable stock or water
2 garlic cloves
salt and freshly ground black pepper

Put the onion into a non-stick pan, cover and cook gently for about 7 minutes, until the onion is tender and lightly browned, stirring from time to time. Add the carrot, lentils and the stock or water, bring to the boil, then reduce the heat, cover and leave to boil gently for 20 minutes, stirring occasionally, until the lentils are pale golden and soft. Put in a food processor or blender with the garlic and whiz until smooth. Return to the saucepan and simmer gently for 3–4 minutes to cook the garlic. Season with salt and freshly ground black pepper.

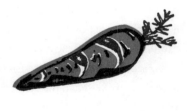

tomato, ginger and chick pea soup

An unusual, delicious and filling soup.

serves 4

Put the onion into a non-stick pan, cover and cook gently for about 7 minutes, until the onion is tender and lightly browned, stirring from time to time. Add the potato, cover and cook gently for 5 minutes, until the vegetables are becoming tender, stirring from time to time to prevent sticking. Add the garlic and ginger; cook for a few seconds, stirring, to cook them lightly, then add the chick peas (garbanzo beans), tomatoes and stock or water. Bring to the boil, then cover, reduce the heat and leave to boil gently for 15–20 minutes, until all the vegetables are tender. Season with salt and freshly ground black pepper.

1 onion, chopped
450g/1lb potatoes, peeled and cut into 1cm/½ in dice
1 large garlic clove, chopped
walnut-sized piece of fresh ginger, chopped
425g/15oz can chick peas (garbanzo beans), drained and rinsed
425g/15oz can tomatoes in juice
600ml/20fl oz/2½ cups vegetable stock or water
salt and freshly ground black pepper

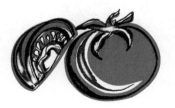

french onion soup

In this soup, the onions are first browned slowly in very little oil, before the stock is added. This long browning process at the beginning is important because it gives this soup its flavour and colour.

serves 4

1tsp olive oil
450g/1lb onions, finely sliced
1tbsp brown rice flour
850ml/30fl oz/3¾ cups vegetable stock or water
salt and freshly ground black pepper
1–2tbsp chopped spring (green) onion or chives, to serve

Heat the oil in a large saucepan, add in the onions, stir, then fry them slowly for 15–20 minutes until they're lightly browned and very tender, stirring often, particularly towards the end of cooking time. Stir in the flour, cook for a few seconds, then pour in the stock or water. Bring to the boil, then let it simmer gently, uncovered, for 10 minutes, to cook the flour. Season with salt and freshly ground black pepper. Serve with a sprinkling of spring (green) onions or chives.

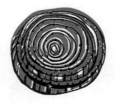

creamy curried parsnip soup

A light curry flavour adds zing to parsnip soup whilst some soya milk gives a creamy texture – a very pleasant combination. Ordinary curry powder is fine for this recipe: use your favourite. I prefer a medium one.

serves 4

1 onion, finely chopped
1 carrot, finely sliced
450g/1lb parsnips, peeled and cut into 1cm/½ in dice
1tbsp curry powder
600ml/20fl oz/2½ cups vegetable stock or water
300ml/10fl oz/1¼ cups soya milk
salt and freshly ground black pepper
1–2tbsp chopped fresh chives, to serve

Put the onion into a non-stick pan, cover and cook gently for about 7 minutes, until the onion is tender and lightly browned, stirring from time to time. Add the carrot and parsnip. Stir, then turn down the heat, cover and leave to cook gently for a further 5 minutes, until the vegetables are getting tender, stirring often to prevent sticking. Stir in the curry powder, cook for a few seconds until it smells aromatic and then add the stock or water. Bring to the boil, reduce the heat, cover and leave to boil gently for about 15 minutes, stirring occasionally, until the vegetables are very tender.

Pour the mixture into a food processor or blender with the soya milk, and whiz until smooth. Return to the saucepan and season with salt and freshly ground black pepper. Reheat gently before serving, but don't let it boil or the soya milk will curdle. Serve each bowlful topped with chopped chives.

mexican black bean soup with tomato salsa

This is a very hearty and filling soup which makes a satisfying meal, especially if you serve it with some wholewheat bread. You can buy the black beans at large supermarkets and health food stores.

serves 4

250g/9oz/1¼ cups dried black beans
1 onion, chopped
1 large carrot, diced
1 celery stalk, diced
1 garlic clove, chopped
2 sprigs of parsley
1 bay leaf
½ tsp cumin seeds
½ tsp ground coriander
1tsp dried oregano
juice of ½ a lemon
salt and freshly ground black pepper

for the tomato salsa
4 tomatoes, chopped
4 spring (green) onions, thinly sliced
small bunch of fresh coriander (cilantro), chopped
juice of ½ a lemon

Put the beans into a large pan with enough water to cover by about 5cm/2 in. Bring to the boil, boil for 1 minute, then remove from the heat and leave to stand for 1 hour.

Add the onion, carrot, celery, garlic, parsley and bay leaf. Bring to the boil. Boil for 5 minutes, then reduce and simmer gently, covered, until the beans are very tender – 1–1½ hours. Add the cumin, ground coriander and oregano. Cook for a further 30 minutes. Remove and discard the parsley stems and bay leaf. Purée about half the beans in a food processor or blender. Put the purée back into the pan. If it is very thick, add a little water to get it to the consistency you like. Reheat gently, add the lemon juice and season with salt and freshly ground black pepper.

Make the salsa by mixing together all the ingredients, season and put into a small bowl. Ladle the soup into bowls and let people spoon the salsa on top of the soup themselves.

butter bean and leek soup with thyme

There's something very satisfying about making this warming, comforting winter soup. If you want to speed the process up, use canned beans instead of dried.

serves 4

Put the beans into a large pan with enough water to cover them by about 5cm/2 in. Bring to the boil, boil for 1 minute, then remove from the heat and leave to stand for 1 hour.

Add the leeks, onion, garlic, thyme and curry powder. Bring to the boil. Boil for 5 minutes, then reduce and simmer gently, covered, until the beans are very tender – 1–1½ hours. Purée the soup in a food processor or blender. Put the purée back in the pan. If it is very thick, add a little water to get it to the consistency you like. Reheat gently and add salt, freshly ground black pepper and enough of the lemon juice to bring out the flavour. Serve sprinkled with chopped parsley.

250g/9oz/1¼ cups dried
butter or lima beans or 2 x
425g/15oz cans
2 leeks, sliced
1 onion, sliced
2 garlic cloves, sliced
½ tsp dried thyme
½ tsp curry powder
salt and freshly ground
black pepper
juice of 1 lemon
1–2tbsp chopped fresh
parsley, to serve

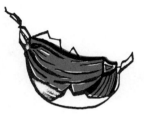

yellow split pea and vegetable soup

This split pea soup originated from Czechoslovakia and is unusual in that it is thickened with a little flour, in addition to the natural thickness which the split peas provide. This gives an interesting texture – a smooth base with tender split peas.

serves 4–6

225g/8oz/heaping 1 cup yellow split peas

2 litres/70fl oz/9 cups water

2 onions, finely chopped

2 carrots, finely sliced

1 garlic clove, crushed

1–2tbsp wholewheat flour

salt and freshly ground black pepper

Put the split peas into a saucepan with the water; let them simmer gently for 40–50 minutes until they're tender, then purée them in a food processor or blender.

Meanwhile, put the onion in a non-stick pan, cover and cook gently for about 7 minutes, until the onion is tender and lightly browned, stirring from time to time. Add the carrot, stir, cover and cook for a further 5 minutes. Stir in the garlic and flour, cook for a minute or two, then gradually pour in the split pea purée, stirring until you have a smooth mixture. Let the soup simmer for 5–10 minutes to cook the flour, then season with salt and freshly ground black pepper. This makes quite a thick soup; if you want it thinner you can always add more liquid.

spanish chick pea soup

Traditionally this would be made with dried chick peas (garbanzo beans) but I've adapted the method and timings for the canned variety. Look out for the organic ones which are now becoming widely available.

serves 4

Put the onion into a non-stick pan, cover and cook gently for about 7 minutes, until the onion is tender and lightly browned, stirring from time to time. Add the potato and carrot, stir, then turn down the heat, cover and leave to cook gently for a further 5 minutes, stirring from time to time to prevent sticking. Add the garlic, stir over the heat for a few seconds to cook it lightly, then add the chick peas (garbanzo beans) and stock or water. Bring to the boil, then add the spinach or cabbage. Bring back to the boil, and leave to boil gently for 15–20 minutes, stirring occasionally. Season with salt and freshly ground black pepper.

1 onion, chopped
1 potato, peeled and cut into 1cm/½ in dice
2 carrots, cut into 5cm/¼ in slices
1 large garlic clove, chopped
425g/15oz can chick peas (garbanzo beans), drained and rinsed
600ml/20fl oz/2½ cups vegetable stock or water
225g/8oz spinach or green cabbage, shredded
salt and freshly ground black pepper

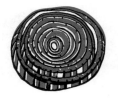

leek, carrot and tarragon soup

A pretty, golden soup flecked with orange and green from the leeks, carrots and tarragon.

serves 4

4 leeks, finely sliced
2 large carrots, cut into 5mm/¼ in dice
850ml/30fl oz/3¾ cups vegetable stock or water
grated nutmeg
salt and freshly ground black pepper
1–2tbsp chopped fresh tarragon, to serve

Put the leek into a non-stick pan, cover and cook gently for about 5 minutes, until it is beginning to soften, stirring from time to time. Add the carrot and the stock or water, bring to the boil, reduce the heat, cover and leave to boil gently for 15–20 minutes, stirring occasionally, until the leeks and carrots are fully cooked. Purée a ladleful of the soup in a food processor or blender, then stir this into the rest of the soup in the saucepan. Season with a little nutmeg, salt and freshly ground black pepper. Serve sprinkled with chopped tarragon.

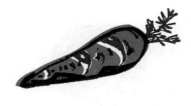

celery, tomato and sweet red pepper soup

This is a delicious, chunky soup. It's good either hot or cold, when it's rather like gazpacho.

serves 4

Put the onion, sweet pepper and celery into a non-stick saucepan and cook, without any additional fat or liquid, for 6–7 minutes, until they are flecked with brown and getting soft, stirring often to prevent sticking. Add the garlic and the tomatoes, chopping them with the spoon once they're in the pan. Add the stock or water. Bring to the boil, reduce the heat, cover and leave to boil gently for 30 minutes, stirring occasionally, until the vegetables are very tender. Purée a generous ladleful of the soup in a food processor or blender, then return it to the rest of the soup and stir. Season with salt and freshly ground black pepper.

1 onion, chopped
2 sweet red peppers, deseeded and chopped
1 head celery, finely sliced
2 large garlic cloves, chopped
425g/15oz can tomatoes in juice
400ml/14fl oz/1¾ cups vegetable stock or water
salt and freshly ground black pepper

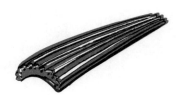

chilled cucumber soup

For a complete change of pace, chilled cucumber soup is very refreshing either as a first course or cooling snack in hot weather.

serves 4

1 cucumber, peeled and cut into rough chunks
425ml/15fl oz/2 cups low-fat plain yogurt
8 sprigs of mint
4 sprigs of parsley
2 spring (green) onions, chopped
1 garlic clove, optional
salt and freshly ground black pepper
4 sprigs of mint and ice cubes to garnish, optional

Put the cucumber into a food processor or blender with the yogurt, mint, parsley, spring (green) onions, and garlic if you're using this, and whiz to a purée. Season with salt and freshly ground black pepper, then serve, garnished with mint and with an ice cube in each bowl if you wish.

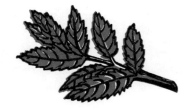

Some tasty dips and spreads are very useful when you're eating a low-fat, low-sugar diet. They take the place of both cheese and butter in sandwiches and on toast, crispbreads and crostini, as well as making tasty first courses and additions to salads.

Many of the savoury dips in this section are based on beans or lentils which make wonderfully flavoursome dips and spreads, thick or thin, smooth or chunky as you prefer. Mix them with fresh herbs, spices, lemon juice, tomato paste, garlic, sweet peppers and other vegetables – there are many possibilities. Tofu, too – well-flavoured, of course – is excellent dip-and-spread material.

Sweet spreads – to replace honey, jam and even chocolate spread – require a little more ingenuity when sugar in any kind of serious quantity is out of bounds. As I've explained in the introduction to this book, I've taken the tough route and even banished fruit, which would be a relatively easy option for sweet spreads and of course there are plenty of no-added sugar preserves, sweetened with fruit juice, available if your diet is more lenient.

But for those who cannot bend the rules this far, I have found several useful sugar replacements: canned chestnut purée (unsweetened, of course); cooked and puréed butternut squash; carob powder, that so-called 'chocolate replacement' usually scorned by chocoholics but usually really appreciated by anyone on a diet which denies the real thing; and fruit teas which provide the flavour of fruit without the sugar.

tofu and fresh herb dip

Tofu needs plenty of flavouring, but with the addition of onion, garlic and herbs it makes a tasty dip.

serves 4

1 small onion, finely chopped
1–2 garlic cloves
8 good sprigs of parsley
285g/10oz packet tofu, drained
salt and freshly ground black pepper

Put the onion into a non-stick pan, cover and cook gently for about 7 minutes, until it is tender and lightly browned, stirring from time to time. Put the onion into a food processor or blender with the garlic and parsley sprigs and whiz until they are well chopped. Cut the tofu into rough chunks and add to the parsley mixture; whiz again until the tofu is blended – you can make it smooth, or leave it a little more lumpy, like fine cottage cheese. Season with salt and freshly ground black pepper.

variation
curried tofu dip

For a spicy alternative, omit the parsley. Instead, stir 2 teaspoons of curry powder into the cooked onion and heat for a few seconds, until it smells aromatic. Continue with the recipe as above, but put 1 teaspoon of tomato paste into the food processor along with the tofu.

tsatsiki

Both the cucumber and the yogurt need to be prepared in advance but after that the dip can be assembled very quickly.

serves 4

Tip the yogurt into a sieve lined with a double layer of kitchen paper. Set over a bowl and leave for 1 hour, by which time the yogurt will be thick. Discard the liquid in the bowl. Also in advance, put the cucumber pieces into a colander, sprinkle with a little salt, place a plate and a weight on top, and leave for about 30 minutes, to remove excess liquid.

Pat the cucumber dry with kitchen paper, then mix with the yogurt, garlic, spring (green) onion and mint. Season with some freshly ground black pepper – it probably won't need any salt.

500g/1lb 2oz carton low-fat plain yogurt
1 large cucumber, peeled and cut into 5mm/¼ in dice
salt
1 garlic clove, crushed
2 spring (green) onions, chopped
2tbsp chopped fresh mint
freshly ground black pepper

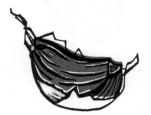

butter bean, sweet red pepper and basil spread

This lovely, brick-red spread is delicious as a dip, spread on toast or crackers or as a topping for baked potatoes.

serves 4

425g/15oz can butter or lima beans
1tbsp freshly-squeezed lemon juice
1 garlic clove, crushed
4 sprigs of basil
1 small sweet red pepper, deseeded and very finely chopped
salt and freshly ground black pepper

Drain and rinse the beans under cold water. Put them into a food processor or blender with the lemon juice, garlic and basil and whiz to a purée. Mix in the sweet pepper and season with salt and freshly ground black pepper.

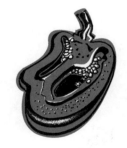

middle-eastern bean pâté

The traditional beans for this are ful medames or dried broad (fava) beans, which you can buy in cans in Middle-Eastern shops. If you can't get them, use a dark, strongly-flavoured bean such as borlotti, or green lentils. This is good as a spread, a dip with crudités, or as part of a salad.

serves 4

Drain and rinse the beans under cold water. Put them into a food processor or blender with the onion, lemon juice, garlic and parsley and whiz to a chunky purée. Add a little water if the mixture needs it, but the aim is to make it quite thick. Season with salt and freshly ground black pepper.

425g/15oz can ful medames beans
a small piece of onion
1tbsp freshly-squeezed lemon juice
1 garlic clove, crushed
1tbsp finely chopped fresh parsley
salt and freshly ground black pepper

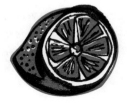

curried tofu and vegetable spread

This is the same tasty tofu mixture which is used in one of the burger recipes and as the base of a flan. I actually invented it originally as a dip to eat with salad or pile on to crispbreads or toast. So here it is in its first form.

serves 4–6

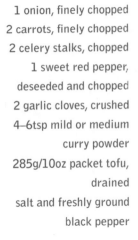

1 onion, finely chopped

2 carrots, finely chopped

2 celery stalks, chopped

1 sweet red pepper, deseeded and chopped

2 garlic cloves, crushed

4–6tsp mild or medium curry powder

285g/10oz packet tofu, drained

salt and freshly ground black pepper

Put the onion into a non-stick pan, cover and cook gently for about 7 minutes, until the onion is tender and lightly browned, stirring from time to time. Add the carrot, celery, sweet pepper and garlic and cook for a further 2–3 minutes, so that the vegetables soften a little but are still very crunchy. Add the curry powder and cook for a further minute. Remove from the heat. Whiz the tofu in a food processor or blender, or mash very well, so that it is smooth-crumbly, like fine cottage cheese. Add this to the curry mixture and season with salt and freshly ground black pepper.

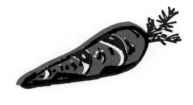

cannellini bean and green herb spread

You can use whatever fresh herbs you fancy in this: parsley makes a good basis, but some other herbs – such as tarragon, dill or basil – are also needed for depth of flavour.

serves 4

Drain and rinse the beans under cold water. Put them into a food processor or blender with the lemon juice, garlic and herbs and whiz to a chunky purée. Add a little water if the mixture needs it, but the aim is to make it quite thick. Season with salt and freshly ground black pepper.

425g/15oz can cannellini beans
1tbsp freshly-squeezed lemon juice
1 garlic clove, crushed
4 sprigs of parsley
4 sprigs of tarragon, dill or basil
salt and freshly ground black pepper

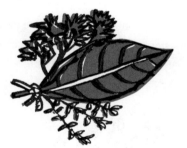

butter bean and tomato spread

This spread is particularly good as a sandwich filling.

serves 4

425g/15oz can butter or lima beans
a small piece of onion
1tbsp freshly-squeezed lemon juice
1tbsp tomato paste
salt and freshly ground black pepper

Drain and rinse the beans under cold water. Put them into a food processor or blender with the onion, lemon juice and tomato paste and whiz to a purée. Season with salt and freshly ground black pepper.

variation

butter bean and mint spread

For this tasty alternative, simply replace the tomato paste with 4 sprigs of mint. This gives a refreshing spread that is particularly good with crisp lettuce.

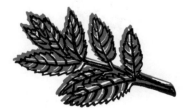

carrot and lemon spread

This spread has a sweet flavour which makes it a good topping for bread, toast or crisp crackers.

serves 1–2

Cover the carrots in boiling water and cook until they are tender. Drain well, reserving a little of the cooking water. Purée the carrots in a food processor or blender until very smooth. Add the lemon rind and juice and little of the reserved cooking water if necessary to make a spreading consistency. If you want to eat this as a sweet spread, don't add any seasoning; if you want it savoury, season with salt and freshly ground black pepper.

225g/8oz carrots, sliced
grated rind and juice of ½ a lemon
salt and freshly ground black pepper

variations

carrot and ginger spread

Prepare as described above, adding ½ a teaspoonful of grated fresh ginger with the lemon. If you prefer a milder taste, cook the ginger with the carrots.

carrot and garlic spread

Add 2 sliced garlic cloves to the carrots along with the water; cook and purée as described above.

carrot and coriander spread

Cook the carrots with 2 sliced garlic cloves; purée as described, then add 1 tablespoon chopped fresh coriander (cilantro). Other fresh herbs such as chopped chives or parsley could be used.

butternut squash and carob spread

Cooked butternut squash has a delicious sweet flavour and creamy texture.

serves 1–2

½ butternut squash, seeds removed

1tsp carob powder

1tsp real vanilla extract

Preheat the oven to 200°C/400°F/gas mark 6.

Put the butternut squash cut-side down on to a baking tray and bake for 45–60 minutes, or until it's tender. Cool, then scoop the flesh away from the skin using a spoon and discard the skin. All this can be done well in advance if convenient.

To make the spread, mash or purée the butternut squash with the carob powder and vanilla extract.

chestnut carob spread

Here is another sweet, chocolatey spread which will go down well with children.

serves 1–2

¼ x 425g/15oz can unsweetened chestnut purée

1tsp carob powder

1tsp real vanilla extract

1—2tbsp water

Blend together the chestnut purée, carob powder and vanilla extract with enough water to make a thick, sweet, chocolatey spread.

blackcurrant jelly preserve

This does not keep in the same way as a normal preserve but in other ways resembles it – it can be used on bread, as a filling for cakes, a topping for desserts, or for serving with savoury dishes.

makes 100g/3¹/₃ oz/ ¹/₃ cup

Put the tea bags into a bowl, pour over the boiling water and leave for at least 30 minutes to infuse. Then squeeze out the tea bags to extract as much of the flavour as possible and discard the tea bags. Put the potato flour (starch) into a small saucepan, mix to a paste with a little of the tea, and then add the rest of the tea. Place over a gentle heat and stir until thickened. Cool and use as required.

4 blackcurrant tea bags
150ml/5fl oz/²/₃ cup boiling water
1tbsp potato flour (starch)

variations

raspberry jelly preserve
Use raspberry tea bags instead of blackcurrant.

orange jelly preserve
Use orange-based tea bags instead of blackcurrant.

salads

Many of the recipes in this section are for fairly substantial salads which will take the place of traditional but fatty salad additions, such as cheese and eggs. (For delicious quiche replacements, see pages 92–94.) These main course salads would be served with leaves, tomatoes, cucumber and other vegetables to make a complete meal – and for these accompaniments I've included in the section some low-fat dressings.

Lighter salads include Tomatoes and Broad Beans with Basil; Broccoli and Sweet Red Pepper Salad; Cucumber, Mustard and Dill Salad and Vegetables à La Grecque which I must say I feel is, along with Leek and Tomato Vinaigrette, a star in the repertoire of low-fat dishes.

bean, tomato and spring onion salad

This is a refreshing yet filling salad with good protein provided by the beans. If you're serving it as a main course, these quantities will serve two.

serves 4

425g/15oz can butter or lima beans
450g/1lb tomatoes, sliced
4 spring (green) onions
1–2tbsp freshly-squeezed lemon juice
salt and freshly ground black pepper

Drain the beans and rinse in cold water. Put them into a bowl with the tomatoes. Chop the spring (green) onions, including the green part, and add to the bowl, along with the lemon juice, a little salt and plenty of freshly ground black pepper. Mix together well.

variation

Instead of lemon juice, use a few tablespoons of Tomato Vinaigrette (page 41) to dress this salad.

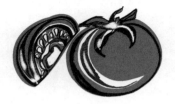

tabbouleh

This simple, very nutritious salad usually has a dressing of olive oil and lemon but is also very good with just the lemon juice. It keeps well and can be made in advance – even overnight – and the ingredients can be varied to your taste. I love this salad served with Yogurt and Fresh Herb Dressing (page 41) and sliced tomatoes, along with cos lettuce leaves for scooping it up and eating it, Lebanese-style.

serves 4

Put the bulgur wheat into a bowl, cover generously with boiling water and leave to soak: 15 minutes for fine bulgur, 2 hours for the coarser type. Drain into a sieve or colander and press with your hands or the back of a spoon to make sure it's as dry as possible. Mix the bulgur with all the remaining ingredients, seasoning well with salt and freshly ground black pepper.

200g/7oz/heaping 1 cup bulgur wheat, preferably fine
1 onion, finely chopped
2 tomatoes, finely chopped
8 spring (green) onions, finely chopped
200g/7oz/3½ cups finely chopped fresh parsley
juice of 1 lemon
salt and freshly ground black pepper

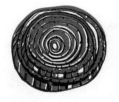

puy lentil salad

I like puy lentils for this salad because they cook quickly, hold their shape well and have a very good flavour. They are available from many supermarkets, but if you can't get them, use the larger green lentils instead. Yogurt and Fresh Herb Dressing (page 41), goes well with this.

serves 4

200g/7oz/1 cup puy lentils
1 bay leaf
1 onion, thinly sliced
1 garlic clove, crushed
1tbsp freshly-squeezed lemon juice
2tbsp chopped fresh parsley
salt and freshly ground black pepper

Put the lentils into a saucepan with the bay leaf and enough water to cover them generously. Bring to the boil, turn down the heat and leave to boil gently until the lentils are tender, about 40–45 minutes. Drain the lentils and put them into a bowl with the onion, garlic, lemon juice and parsley. Season with salt and freshly ground black pepper and mix well. Serve hot, warm or cool. The salad improves if left to stand for at least an hour to allow the flavours to develop.

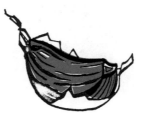

black bean and ginger salad with lime

Black beans have a delicious flavour and mealy texture. You can buy the dried beans in large supermarkets and health food stores.

serves 4

Cover the dried beans with cold water and soak overnight or for 6–8 hours, or cover them with cold water, bring to the boil, boil for 2–3 minutes, then leave to stand for 1 hour.

Put the beans, ginger and garlic into a large saucepan with the water, bring to the boil, then leave to boil gently, uncovered, for 1 hour, until the beans are very tender. Drain off the excess water. Put the beans into a bowl with the lime rind and juice, the spring (green) onions and sesame oil – as much or as little as you wish. Season with salt and freshly ground black pepper and mix well. Serve warm or cold. The salad improves if left to stand for at least an hour to allow the flavours to develop.

200g/7oz/1 cup dried black beans
2 walnut-sized pieces of fresh ginger, chopped
3 large garlic cloves, chopped
1.75 litres/60fl oz/7 ½ cups water
grated rind and juice of 1 lime
bunch of spring (green) onions, chopped
sesame oil
salt and freshly ground black pepper

tomatoes with broad beans and basil

I think broad (fava) beans are a very under-valued vegetable. Frozen ones are tiny and tender, but if you don't like the skins, simply pop the beans out of them after cooking – their vivid green looks very pretty with the red tomato and basil.

serves 4

450g/1lb/heaping 2 cups frozen broad (fava) beans
450g/1lb tomatoes, sliced
8 large basil leaves, torn
1–2tbsp freshly-squeezed lemon juice
salt and freshly ground black pepper

Cook the broad beans in a little fast-boiling water until just tender, then drain and cool. When the beans are cool enough to handle, pop off the grey outer skins, if you wish. Mix the beans with the tomatoes, basil and some lemon juice, salt and freshly ground black pepper.

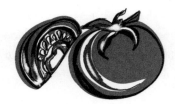

lemony bean salad with tarragon

Lemon and tarragon add a lovely zingy flavour to this simple salad. You can soak and cook dried beans for this recipe or use canned ones.

serves 4

Cover the dried beans with cold water and soak overnight or for 6–8 hours, or cover them with cold water, bring to the boil, boil for 2–3 minutes, then leave to stand for 1 hour.

Put the soaked beans into a large saucepan with the water and garlic, bring to the boil, then leave to boil gently, uncovered, for 1 hour, until the beans are very tender. Drain off the excess water. If you're using canned beans, drain them and rinse in cold water.

Put the beans into a bowl with the lemon rind and juice and tarragon. Season with salt and freshly ground black pepper and mix gently. Serve warm or cold. The salad improves if left to stand for at least an hour to allow the flavours to develop.

200g/7oz/1 cup dried cannellini beans or 2 x 425g/15oz cans cannellini beans
1.75 litres/60fl oz/7½ cups water
3 large garlic cloves, chopped
grated rind and juice of 1 lemon
2 good tbsp chopped fresh tarragon
salt and freshly ground black pepper

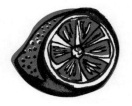

grilled sweet pepper, spinach and puy lentil salad

Very nutritious and a great combination of flavours, colours and textures. You can cook the lentils yourself or buy them in cans. Yogurt and Fresh Herb Dressing (page 41) goes well with this salad.

serves 4

200g/7oz/1 cup puy lentils
or 2 x 425g/15oz cans
squeeze of lemon juice
salt and freshly ground
black pepper
2 sweet red peppers
250g/8oz/4 cups young
spinach
lemon wedges

First deal with the lentils. If you're using dried ones, put them into a saucepan with a generous covering of water and bring to the boil. Cover, then boil gently for 40–45 minutes, or until they are tender; drain. For canned lentils, just drain and rinse in cold water. Season the lentils with salt, freshly ground black pepper and a squeeze of lemon juice.

Meanwhile, prepare the peppers by halving them and removing the core and seeds. Put the halves, rounded-side up, on a baking tray and put under a hot grill (broiler) for 10–15 minutes, or until the peppers are tender and the skin blackened in places. When they have cooled a little, you can remove the papery skins if you wish, or leave them on – I prefer them on. Cut the peppers into strips.

Prepare the spinach by cooking it in a dry saucepan for a minute or two until it has wilted – get it as tender as you want it, then drain off the liquid and season with salt, freshly ground black pepper and lemon juice. Arrange the peppers, lentils and spinach on individual plates or in a serving dish, garnished with some lemon wedges.

leek and tomato vinaigrette

This dish of leeks – cooked until tender and then marinated in a simple tomato dressing – makes an excellent first course or can be served as a salad along with some green salad leaves.

serves 4

Cut the leeks into 8–10cm/3–4 in lengths, then cook in boiling water until really tender, about 7–10 minutes. Drain the leeks and put them into a shallow dish. Mix together the tomato juice and lemon juice, then pour over the leeks, moving them around to make sure they are all well coated. Season with salt and freshly ground black pepper. Leave for 1 hour if possible, to allow the flavours to blend, then sprinkle the chives on top and serve.

6 leeks
150ml/5fl oz/⅔ cup tomato juice
1tbsp freshly-squeezed lemon juice
salt and freshly ground black pepper
1tbsp finely chopped fresh chives

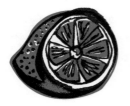

vegetables à la grecque

Many vegetables are suitable for this dish; I've used French (fine green) beans, cauliflower and courgettes (zucchini), but you could try it with tender young carrots and turnips, spring (green) onions, broccoli and fennel, for instance.

serves 4

225g/8oz French (fine green) beans, cut into 2.5cm/1 in lengths
1 small cauliflower, divided into florets
2 courgettes (zucchini), sliced
150ml/5fl oz/⅔ cup tomato juice
1tbsp coriander seeds, roughly crushed
2 bay leaves
1 garlic clove, crushed
2tbsp freshly-squeezed lemon juice
salt and freshly ground black pepper
1–2tbsp chopped fresh parsley or coriander (cilantro)

Cook the French (fine green) beans, cauliflower and courgettes (zucchini) in boiling water until they are just tender when tested with the point of a knife. If you're careful, you might be able to do them all together, in a large pan in 5cm/2 in of water, or it might be easier to do them in separate batches, to make sure none of them get overcooked. In any case, put the boiled vegetables into a shallow dish.

Put the tomato juice into a pan with the coriander seeds, bay leaves and garlic and bring to the boil. Add the lemon juice, and pour this mixture over the vegetables, moving them around to make sure they are all well-coated. Season with salt and freshly ground black pepper. Leave for 1 hour, to allow the flavours to develop and blend, then sprinkle the fresh parsley or coriander (cilantro) on top and serve.

cucumber, mustard and dill salad

This is a very refreshing salad which needs to be made in advance. Cover it well, then drain it at the last minute, just before you serve it.

serves 2–4

Mix all the ingredients together and leave for at least an hour (overnight is fine), to draw the juices out the cucumber. Drain the salad just before serving, discarding the liquid. Check the seasoning, and serve.

1 cucumber, peeled and thinly sliced
2 large spring (green) onions, sliced
1tsp whole mustard seeds
4 sprigs of fresh dill, chopped
2tbsp freshly-squeezed lemon juice
salt and freshly ground black pepper

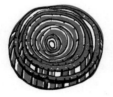

broccoli and sweet red pepper salad

The combination of lightly cooked broccoli and grilled (broiled) sweet pepper makes a very pleasant salad and one that doesn't call for oily dressings to enhance the fresh flavours, just a squeeze of lemon juice and some salt and freshly ground black pepper.

serves 2

2 sweet red peppers
250g/9oz broccoli
salt and freshly ground black pepper
squeeze of lemon juice

First prepare the peppers. Cut them in half, remove the core and seeds and put the halves, rounded-side up, on a baking tray or grill (broiler) pan. Cook under a hot grill (broiler) for 10–15 minutes, or until the peppers are tender and the skin blackened in places. When they have cooled a little, you can remove the papery skins if you wish, or leave them on – I prefer them on. Cut the peppers into strips.

Meanwhile, cook the broccoli. Cut it into even-sized, smallish florets and use any of the stem that seems fairly tender too. Cook in 1cm/½ in fast-boiling water, covered, for about 5 minutes, or until tender but not soggy. Drain and refresh in cold running water; drain again.

Mix together the pepper strips and broccoli florets and season with salt, freshly ground black pepper and a squeeze of lemon juice.

potato salad with chives and dill

The secret of a good potato salad is to cook the potatoes until they're just tender. The potatoes need to be firm, and of course using a waxy type – such as new potatoes – also helps to achieve this. You don't need loads of oil or mayonnaise to make a good potato salad: some low-fat yogurt and chopped fresh herbs makes a delicious dressing.

serves 4

Cook the potatoes, whole if small otherwise cut into even-sized pieces, in boiling salted water until they are just tender – probably around 15 minutes, but keep an eye on them because the little ones cook quickly. Drain and put into a bowl with the yogurt, salt and freshly ground black pepper and the herbs. Mix gently, then leave to cool.

700g/1½ lb waxy potatoes, scrubbed
150ml/5fl oz/ ⅔ cup low-fat plain yogurt
salt and freshly ground black pepper
1tbsp chopped fresh chives
1tbsp chopped fresh dill

variation

Some chopped spring (green) onion – white and green parts – is a pleasant addition.

beetroot with dill dressing

The sweet tenderness of beetroot (beet) is enhanced by a sharp yogurt and fresh dill dressing. Use ready-cooked beetroots (beets) if you can find ones which have not been prepared with vinegar; otherwise, buy raw ones and cook them yourself.

serves 4

4 beetroots (beets)
150ml/5fl oz/⅔ cup low-fat plain yogurt
1tbsp chopped fresh dill
1tbsp freshly-squeezed lemon juice
salt and freshly ground black pepper

If the beetroots (beets) are raw, put them into a saucepan, cover with cold water, bring to the boil, cover the pan and boil gently for 1–1½ hours or a little longer if necessary, until they are tender right through to the middle when tested with a skewer or sharp knife. (If you have a pressure cooker, this time can be reduced to about 30 minutes.) Drain, cool a little, then slip off the skins.

Slice the beetroot (beets) into quite thin rounds and put these on to a serving dish. Mix together the yogurt, dill and lemon juice and season with salt and freshly ground black pepper. Pour this over the beetroot (beets) and serve.

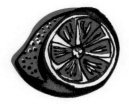

dressings

yogurt and fresh herb dressing

Mix all the ingredients together, seasoning to taste with salt and freshly ground black pepper.

150ml/5fl oz/⅔ cup low-fat plain yogurt
1tbsp chopped fresh parsley
1tbsp chopped fresh tarragon, dill, chives or basil
1tbsp freshly-squeezed lemon juice
salt and freshly ground black pepper

whole mustard dressing

Mix all the ingredients together, seasoning to taste with salt and freshly ground black pepper. Stir before using.

1tsp wholegrain mustard
juice of 1 lemon
2tbsp water
salt and freshly ground black pepper

tomato vinaigrette

I find this a very useful fat-free dressing; it's tasty and coats leaves well.

Mix all the ingredients together, seasoning to taste with salt and freshly ground black pepper.

150ml/5fl oz/⅔ cup pure tomato juice
1tbsp freshly-squeezed lemon juice
1 small garlic clove, crushed, optional
salt and freshly ground black pepper

variation

tomato and herb vinaigrette
Add 1–2 tablespoons chopped fresh chives or basil to the dressing.

All the dishes in this section can be made on top of the stove and they're all easy to do. Most of them are one-pot meals that require little in the way of accompaniments, although cooked grains – rice of course, or millet or quinoa for something a little different – complement them and soak up the delicious juices.

Many of the dishes begin with the dry-frying of an onion or other vegetables and spices. This is simple and gives lovely flavour to the dish, although it does mean keeping a close watch on the pan. Once the initial frying is done and the rest of the ingredients have been added, most of these dishes can be left to cook without any further attention until they're ready and filling the kitchen with their mouth-watering aroma.

stews and casseroles

cannellini bean stew

A delicious, easy-to-make stew, full of pretty golden colours and the sweet flavours of carrots, parsnips and sweetcorn. Use sweetcorn that has been canned without salt or sugar, and if you can find organic canned tomatoes, they're particularly good.

serves 4

2 onions, chopped
2 celery stalks, sliced
4 leeks, sliced
1 large parsnip, peeled and sliced
225g/8oz carrots, diced
2–3 garlic cloves, chopped
425g/15oz can cannellini beans
325g/11oz can sweetcorn, drained
425g/15oz can tomatoes in juice
300ml/10fl oz/1¼ cups tomato juice
salt and freshly ground black pepper
chopped fresh parsley, to serve

Put the onion into a non-stick saucepan and cook, without any additional fat or liquid, for 6–7 minutes, until it is flecked with brown, stirring it often to prevent sticking. Add the celery, leeks, parsnips, carrots and garlic; stir, then cover again and cook over a gentle heat for a further 5 minutes, until all the vegetables are softening. Keep an eye on them and stir often to prevent sticking.

Drain the cannellini beans and rinse in a sieve under cold water, then add to the pan, along with the sweetcorn, tomatoes and tomato juice. Mash the tomatoes with the spoon to break them up a bit. Bring to the boil, cover, turn down the heat and leave to simmer for a further 20–30 minutes, until all the vegetables are tender. Season with salt and freshly ground black pepper. Sprinkle with chopped parsley before serving.

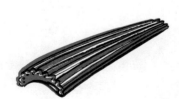

vegetable dal with fresh tomato chutney

Dal is especially good, made in advance and then reheated, as this gives the flavours time to develop. This is delicious just as it is, or can be served with new or baked potatoes. For a real feast, try serving it with brown rice and extra vegetables such as cauliflower and green beans.

serves 3–4

Put the lentils into a saucepan with the onion, garlic, bay leaf, ginger, turmeric and water. Bring to the boil, then turn down the heat and leave to boil gently, uncovered, for 30–40 minutes, or until the lentils are very soft and the mixture is quite thick. There will be some froth on the water at first but don't worry about this; just stir the mixture and it will disappear as the lentils cook. Stir often towards the end of the cooking time to prevent sticking. When the lentils are thick and soft, stir in the cumin and ground coriander and season with salt and freshly ground black pepper.

While the dal is cooking, prepare the vegetables. Bring 1cm/½ in of water to the boil. Put in the cauliflower and beans, bring back to the boil, cover and cook for 5–6 minutes, or until the vegetables are tender. Drain and add the vegetables to the dal. Stir gently and check the seasoning.

Mix together the ingredients for the chutney and serve with the dal.

200g/7oz/1 cup split red lentils
1 onion, chopped
1 large garlic clove, sliced
1 bay leaf
2 thin slices of fresh ginger
½ tsp ground turmeric
1 litre/35fl oz/4½ cups water
1tsp ground cumin
2tsp ground coriander
salt and freshly ground black pepper
225g/8oz cauliflower florets
225g/8oz green beans halved

for the tomato chutney
225g/8oz tomatoes, sliced or chopped
1 small onion or spring (green) onion, sliced
3tbsp chopped fresh coriander (cilantro)

potato casserole

This is a lovely potato casserole based on a traditional Austrian paprikas, or stew. It's not a one-pot stew; I find it best to cook the potatoes before mixing them with the other ingredients, otherwise the acid from the tomato paste can stop them from softening properly. You can peel the potatoes or keep them in their skins, whichever you prefer.

serves 2

450g/1lb potatoes, cut into 2.5cm/1 in pieces
2 onions, sliced
2 garlic cloves, sliced
½ tsp dried oregano
1tsp ground cumin
1tsp ground coriander
300ml/10fl oz/1¼ cups vegetable stock or water
3tbsp tomato paste
salt and freshly ground black pepper

Cover the potatoes in boiling water and cook until they are just tender; drain and set aside. (The cooking water makes good stock for this recipe.) Put the onion into a non-stick saucepan and cook, without any additional fat or liquid, for 6–7 minutes, until it is flecked with brown and getting soft, stirring often to prevent sticking. Add the garlic, oregano, cumin and coriander. Stir over the heat for a few seconds until they smell aromatic. Pour in the stock or water and add the tomato paste and drained potatoes. Stir well, bring to the boil, then reduce the heat and leave to cook gently for 30 minutes, until the sauce is thick and glossy. Season with salt and freshly ground black pepper.

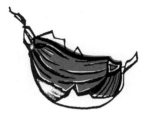

red bean chilli

Serve this chilli with brown rice, quinoa or baked potatoes. If you can't eat very hot foods, you can omit the chilli powder without spoiling the dish, despite the name.

serves 4

Put the onion into a non-stick saucepan and cook, without any additional fat or liquid, for 6–7 minutes, until it is flecked with brown, stirring it often to prevent sticking. Add the garlic, carrot and sweet pepper. Stir, then cover and leave to cook over a gentle heat for 4–5 minutes, stirring occasionally. Add the tomatoes, breaking them up with the spoon when they're in the pan, and the chilli powder, if you're using it.

   Drain the red kidney beans and rinse in cold water, then add to the pan. Bring to the boil, reduce the heat and boil gently for about 20 minutes, until the vegetables are tender and the chilli is thick, stirring from time to time. Season with salt and freshly ground black pepper.

2 onions, finely chopped
2 garlic cloves, crushed
1 large carrot, grated
1 sweet red pepper, deseeded and chopped
425g/15oz can tomatoes in juice
½ tsp hot chilli powder, optional
2 x 425g/15oz cans red kidney beans
salt and freshly ground black pepper

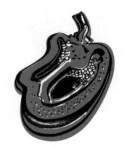

spinach dal

Delicious and packed with iron and nutrients, this dal is excellent on its own or with extras such as potatoes, brown rice and cauliflower. Chard, that relative to spinach with thick ribbed stems, is equally good for this recipe – cut it up, stems and all, and use in exactly the same way.

serves 3

1 litre/35fl oz/4½ cups water
½ tsp ground turmeric
60g/2oz/heaping ¼ cup whole green lentils
125g/4oz/heaping ½ cup split red lentils
500g/1lb 2oz spinach leaves
1 onion, chopped
1 large garlic clove, sliced
1tsp ground cumin
2tsp ground coriander
salt and freshly ground black pepper

Put the water and turmeric into a large saucepan, bring to the boil and add the green lentils. Bring back to the boil and leave to boil, uncovered, for 20 minutes. Add the red lentils and cook for a further 10 minutes, then add the spinach, onion and garlic. Boil gently, uncovered, for a further 10 minutes, until the lentils are very soft, the spinach is tender and the mixture is quite thick. Stir in the cumin and coriander, season with salt and freshly ground black pepper and serve.

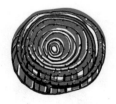

butter bean curry

This curry is particularly good served with cooked brown Basmati rice and Fresh Tomato Chutney (page 45).

serves 4

Put the onion into a non-stick saucepan and cook, without any additional fat or liquid, for 6–7 minutes, until it is flecked with brown, stirring it often to prevent sticking. Add the garlic, ginger, cumin, coriander, cloves and cinnamon stick and stir over the heat for a few seconds until they smell aromatic. Stir in the rice flour and water and bring to the boil, stirring often until slightly thickened.

Drain the butter or lima beans, rinse in cold water and add to the spice mixture, along with the tomatoes. Bring back to the boil and boil gently for 10 minutes. Season with salt and freshly ground black pepper, remove the cinnamon stick and serve.

1 large onion, finely chopped
2 garlic cloves, crushed
2tsp grated fresh ginger
1tsp ground cumin
2tsp ground coriander
2 cloves
5cm/2in piece of cinnamon stick
2tbsp brown rice flour
600ml/20fl oz/2½ cups water
2 x 425g/15oz cans butter or lima beans
4 tomatoes, peeled and chopped
salt and freshly ground black pepper

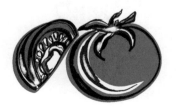

refried red beans

This is low in fat in spite of its name, and is delicious with a mixed salad.

serves 2

1 onion, finely chopped
425g/15oz can red kidney beans
2 tomatoes, peeled and chopped
1 garlic clove, crushed
salt and freshly ground black pepper
1tbsp chopped fresh coriander (cilantro), to serve

Put the onion into a non-stick saucepan and cook, without any additional fat or liquid, for 6–7 minutes, until it is flecked with brown, stirring it often to prevent sticking.

Meanwhile, drain the beans, rinse in cold water and mash roughly with a fork, to give a chunky texture. Add the beans to the onion mixture, together with the tomatoes and garlic. Cook gently, stirring, until everything is heated through. Season with salt and freshly ground black pepper. Serve sprinkled with chopped fresh coriander (cilantro).

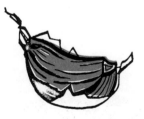

spicy lentil and root vegetable stew

Simple, cheap and warming, this is good served with crunchy-cooked baked potatoes or even healthy chips.

serves 4

Put the onion into a non-stick saucepan and cook, without any additional fat or liquid, for 6–7 minutes, until it is flecked with brown, stirring it often to prevent sticking. Add the garlic, cumin and ground coriander, stir over the heat for a few seconds until the spices smell aromatic, then stir in the casserole vegetables, lentils and the stock or water. Bring to the boil, reduce the heat, cover and leave to boil gently for 20 minutes, stirring occasionally, until the vegetables are tender and the lentils are pale golden and soft.

Add the frozen peas and cook for a few more minutes to heat them through, then season with salt and freshly ground black pepper and serve, sprinkled with fresh coriander (cilantro) if you're using this.

1 onion, chopped
1 garlic clove, crushed
1tsp ground cumin
2tsp ground coriander
450g/1lb mixed prepared casserole vegetables
175g/6oz/scant 1 cup lentils
850ml/30fl oz/3¾ cups vegetable stock or water
125g/4oz/1 cup frozen peas
salt and freshly ground black pepper
2tbsp chopped fresh coriander (cilantro), optional

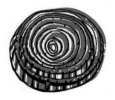

mixed vegetable curry

Don't be put off by the number of ingredients in this recipe; it's very easy to make and delicious served with brown Basmati rice. If there's any left over, it's even better the next day. In fact it can stand several reheatings and tastes better each time but keep it well-covered in the refrigerator in between whiles, particularly if you are on a diet to combat Candida albicans.

serves 4–6

2 onions, finely chopped
4 garlic cloves, crushed
1tsp white mustard seed
4tsp ground turmeric
2tbsp ground coriander
14–16 curry leaves or
½ tsp curry powder
4cm/1½ in piece fresh
ginger, grated
750g/1½ lb potatoes,
scrubbed and cut into 1cm/
½ in pieces
1 large cauliflower, cut
into florets
125g/4oz green beans,
trimmed and halved
2 large carrots, cut into
5mm/¼ in slices
8 spinach or cabbage
leaves, roughly shredded
200ml/7fl oz/¾ cup water
salt and freshly ground
black pepper

Put the onion into a non-stick saucepan and cook, without any additional fat or liquid, for 6–7 minutes, until it is flecked with brown, stirring it often to prevent sticking. Add the garlic and all the spices and stir over the heat for a few seconds until they smell aromatic. Add all the vegetables and stir so that they all get coated with the spices. Pour in the water and bring to the boil. Cover and cook gently for 15–20 minutes, or until the vegetables are just tender and most of the liquid has been absorbed. Season with salt and freshly ground black pepper and serve.

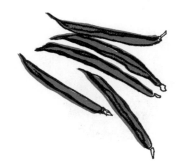

kale dal

I've adapted this recipe from one of Colin Spencer's. It's incredibly healthy and a wonderful way of eating nutritious kale or, indeed, spring greens, which can be used if you can't get kale. I love this with some Fresh Tomato Chutney (page 45) on the side.

serves 3

Put the mustard seeds into a large saucepan and dry-fry for a minute or so until they start to pop. Add the cumin, coriander and turmeric and stir over the heat for a few seconds until they smell aromatic – take care not to burn them. Add the garlic, stock, kale, potatoes and lentils. Bring to the boil, cover and boil gently for 35 minutes, until the lentils are cooked and the potatoes tender. Add the lemon juice and rind and season with salt and freshly ground black pepper.

1tbsp mustard seeds
2tsp ground cumin
2tsp ground coriander
2tsp turmeric
5 garlic cloves, sliced
850ml /30fl oz/3¾ cups
vegetable stock
450g/1lb kale, finely
chopped
450g/1lb potatoes, peeled
and cut into 2.5cm/1 in
pieces
125g/4oz/heaping ½ cup
dry green or brown lentils
grated rind and juice of
1 lemon
salt and freshly ground
black pepper

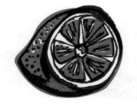

spiced vegetables

This is a lovely dish, lightly spiced but not hot. Serve with Dal Sauce (page 137) or some cooked brown rice, quinoa or millet.

serves 4

1 onion, finely chopped
1 large clove garlic, crushed
1tsp turmeric
1tsp ground coriander
1tsp ground cumin
1 bay leaf
2 carrots, thinly sliced
450g/1lb potatoes, peeled and cut into 1cm/½ in dice
2 leeks, sliced
150ml/5fl oz/⅔ cup water
salt and freshly ground black pepper

Put the onion into a non-stick saucepan and cook, without any additional fat or liquid, for 6–7 minutes, until it is flecked with brown, stirring it often to prevent sticking. Add the garlic, spices and bay leaf and stir over the heat for a few seconds until it smells aromatic. Add the remaining vegetables and stir over the heat for a further 1–2 minutes so that they are all coated with the oil and spices. Add the water and a little salt and freshly ground black pepper. Cover and leave to simmer for 15–20 minutes, until the vegetables are tender, stirring from time to time.

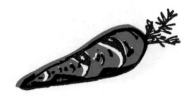

sri lankan curry

This is really easy to make and delicious to eat. I've adapted it a bit by using soya milk instead of coconut milk, which is very high in fat. If you want some coconut flavour, bring the soya milk to the boil with 50g/2oz/²/₃ cup desiccated (shredded) coconut, remove from the heat, cover and leave to infuse for 30 minutes, then strain the milk and discard the coconut. This does add a little fat along with the flavour, but not a lot.

serves 3–4

Put the onion into a non-stick saucepan and cook, without any additional fat or liquid, for 6–7 minutes, until it is flecked with brown, stirring it often to prevent sticking. Add the garlic, stir over the heat for a few seconds and then add the sweet pepper, courgette (zucchini) and curry paste. Stir well, then pour in the soya milk. Bring to the boil, turn down the heat, cover and leave to cook very gently for about 10 minutes, until the vegetables are tender. Stir in the lemon juice, season with salt and freshly ground black pepper, sprinkle with fresh coriander (cilantro) and serve.

1 onion, finely chopped
2 garlic cloves, crushed
1 sweet red pepper, deseeded and chopped
4 courgettes (zucchini), sliced
2tsp curry paste
400ml/14fl oz/1¾ cups soya milk
juice of ½ a lemon
salt and freshly ground black pepper
1tbsp chopped fresh coriander (cilantro), to serve

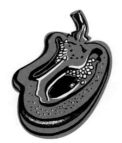

butter beans in creamy sauce

Butter, lima or cannellini beans can be used in this simple recipe. Cooked green vegetables or salad goes well with it.

serves 2

425g/15oz can butter, lima or cannellini beans
2 quantities of Onion Sauce, page 138
grated rind and juice of ½ a lemon
2 good tbsp chopped fresh parsley
salt and freshly ground black pepper

Drain and rinse the beans and put into a saucepan with the onion sauce, lemon juice and parsley. Heat gently, season with salt and freshly ground black pepper and serve.

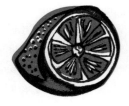

root vegetables in turmeric sauce

This is a beautiful dish of orange and golden root vegetables, bathed in a creamy, delicately flavoured sauce. You could save time by using ready-prepared or frozen root vegetables, sometimes called 'casserole vegetables'.

serves 6

Put the onion into a non-stick saucepan and cook, without any additional fat or liquid, for 6–7 minutes, until it is flecked with brown, stirring it often to prevent sticking. Add the garlic, ginger and turmeric and stir over the heat for a few seconds until the spices smell aromatic. Add all the vegetables and stir well. Pour in the soya milk and bring to the boil. Turn down the heat, cover and leave to cook very gently for about 15–20 minutes, until the vegetables feel tender when pierced with the point of a knife. Season with salt and freshly ground black pepper and serve.

1 onion, chopped
1 garlic clove, crushed
1tsp grated fresh ginger
1tsp turmeric
225g/8oz carrots, cut into
1cm/½ in dice
225g/8oz swede, cut into
1cm/½ in dice
225g/8oz parsnip, cut into
1cm/½ in dice
½ sweet red pepper,
deseeded and sliced
400ml/14fl oz/1¾ cups soya
milk
salt and freshly ground
black pepper

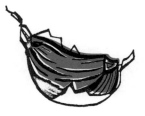

All grains are low-fat, low-sugar ingredients but, as I have explained in the introduction, because of the effect of refined grains on blood-sugar levels, only whole grains feature in the recipes in this book. In fact, whole grains are a valuable food and one which I feel we could make more use of in our meals. They are incredibly easy to cook (as easy as pasta, though generally not as quick to cook), yet they are so rarely used compared to pasta. Rice and the less-well known millet and quinoa make perfect accompaniments to the recipes in the previous section and supply valuable vitamins and minerals, as well as being ideal for mopping up the delicious juices.

Of course grains can also be made into filling, satisfying main dishes in their own right and there are a number of recipes for these in this section too.

brown rice

To cook brown rice, begin by putting the rice into a sieve and rinsing it in cold running water. Then put the rice into a saucepan with two to two and a half times its volume in cold water: 1 cup of rice to 2–2½ cups of water. It's easier to measure it by volume than by weight. The larger amount of water gives a softer grain at the end of cooking, if you continue to cook the rice until all the water has been absorbed. This softness may not be fashionable, but can be very comforting – the choice is yours. Bring the mixture to the boil, then turn the heat right down, cover the pan with a lid and leave the rice to cook for 40–45 minutes, until all the water has been absorbed and the rice is tender. The rice improves if you take it off the heat and leave it to stand, still covered, for 10 minutes after cooking. You could even put a clean folded tea towel under the lid of the pan to help absorb any residual moisture. This method works for long grain, short grain and Basmati brown rice, though brown Basmati only takes 25 minutes to cook.

The other way to cook brown rice is to do it exactly like pasta: bring a large saucepan of water to a rolling boil, add the rice and let it boil until it is tender, about 30–40 minutes for long and short grain, 15–20 minutes for brown Basmati. Then drain the rice into a sieve or colander and pour a kettleful of boiling water over to rinse it.

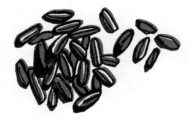

bulgur wheat

Bulgur wheat is the healthy version of couscous, which is a refined wheat product. Bulgur is just as good to eat as couscous, more health-giving and just as easy to prepare. In fact it's easier in some ways because it doesn't go lumpy.

You can buy fine or coarse bulgur wheat. The fine one is quicker to prepare; all you do is soak it in boiling water for 15 minutes, drain off any excess water and it's ready to use. You could then warm it through in a saucepan or, better still, in a steamer for a few minutes, before seasoning and serving. Coarse bulgur needs longer soaking (though as it's already been cooked, it's perfectly all right to eat after a short soak – just rather chewy). Cover it with boiling water and soak for 2 hours; or let it soak in cold water for 4–5 hours, or even overnight. Drain thoroughly and use it as it is, or heat it in the same way as fine bulgur. You can also use bulgur wheat to make a pilaf, exactly as you would use rice, millet or any of the other grains.

millet

Another nutritious grain, millet is the richest in iron and higher in protein than wheat and rice. It's nicest if you toast it in a dry saucepan before adding any water. For the fluffiest, tasty millet it's worth taking the time to toast and soak the millet before cooking it.

To make millet for 2 people, put 125g/4oz/⅔ cup millet into a saucepan, set over a moderate heat and stir for 2–3 minutes, until the millet smells toasted and starts to jump around. Then, standing well back, add 450ml/16fl oz/2 cups of boiling water. Leave to soak for 1 hour, then bring to the boil, cover the pan and leave to boil gently for 40–45 minutes. Turn off the heat and leave the millet to stand for a further 10–15 minutes before fluffing it up with a fork.

quinoa

Pronounced 'keen-wah', quinoa is a particularly nutritious high-protein seed which is cooked and used as a grain. It cooks quickly and is excellent as an accompaniment to bean and lentil dishes or as a main course in its own right with vegetables or salad.

There are two keys to preparing quinoa: wash it thoroughly before cooking, and don't over-cook it.

The reason for the careful washing is that the grains are naturally coated with a substance called saponin which is slightly bitter. Put the quinoa into a bowl of cold water, swish the grains around thoroughly, and repeat the process a couple of times. Then put the quinoa into a sieve and run some cold water through it to be extra sure; drain well.

Bring 1 litre/35fl oz/4½ cups of water to the boil and add the quinoa. Bring back to the boil then start timing: cook for 12 minutes, then check to see if a grain is tender with its white tail showing. If not, cook for a further 2–3 minutes. Drain into a sieve, then put back into the dry saucepan until you're ready to serve it. Season with salt and pepper, some crushed garlic, chopped herbs or grated ginger as desired.

celery rice

A delicious way of using some of the outer (but not too tough) celery stalks, which become buttery-tender and enhance the tomatoey rice.

serves 5–6

2 large onions, chopped
8 celery stalks, sliced
2 sweet red peppers, deseeded and chopped
2 garlic cloves, crushed
350g/12oz/1¾ cups brown rice
425g/15oz can tomatoes in juice
1 litre/35fl oz/4½ cups water
salt and freshly ground black pepper
2tbsp chopped fresh parsley, to serve

Put the onion into a non-stick saucepan and cook, without any additional fat or liquid, for 6–7 minutes, until it is flecked with brown, stirring it often to prevent sticking. Add the celery and sweet pepper. Stir, cover and leave to cook over a gentle heat for 10 minutes, stirring occasionally. Add the garlic, stir over the heat for a few seconds until it smells aromatic and then add the rice. Mix well and add the tomatoes, water and some salt. Bring to the boil and let the mixture simmer away, uncovered, for 40 minutes, until the rice is just about tender and nearly all the water has been absorbed. Take the pan off the heat, cover, and leave to stand, so that the rice can finish cooking in its own steam, for a further 10–15 minutes. Fluff up the mixture with a fork, add freshly ground black pepper to taste and more salt if necessary, and serve sprinkled with the chopped parsley.

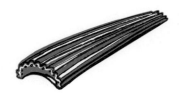

bulgur wheat pilaf

Serve this pilaf with Yogurt and Fresh Herb Dressing (page 41) and a simple tomato salad.

serves 3–4

Put the bulgur wheat and boiling water into a large bowl or saucepan, cover and leave on one side for 15 minutes; it will absorb the water and swell up. Put the onion and sweet pepper into a non-stick saucepan and cook, without any additional fat or liquid, for 6–7 minutes, until they are flecked with brown, stirring often to prevent sticking. Add the garlic and stir over the heat for a few seconds more. Add the bulgar wheat and season with salt and freshly ground black pepper. Cook over a low heat for 5–10 minutes to heat through. Serve sprinkled with the chopped parsley.

225g/8oz/1⅓ cups bulgur wheat
600ml/20fl oz/2½ cups boiling water
2 onions, finely chopped
1 sweet red pepper, deseeded and chopped
1–2 garlic cloves, crushed
salt and freshly ground black pepper
2tbsp chopped fresh parsley, to serve

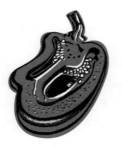

ginger rice with japanese vegetables

This rice dish is exquisite, far more delicate than the amount of ginger might lead you to think. Many Japanese dishes are tasty and very low in fat but often contain sugar in one form or another. In addition, many are flavoured with soy sauce, which is fermented. So this recipe is an adaptation which omits sugar and mirin, the sweet fortified wine with which it would traditionally be flavoured, and uses lemon juice instead of soy sauce. The ajitsuki nori — powdered seaweed — gives a Japanese flavour and can be bought at Chinese or Japanese shops. If you can't get it, just use some chopped fresh parsley. You should use brown rice for this dish.

serves 2

175g/6oz/scant 1 cup rice
50g/2oz/4 in piece fresh ginger, finely chopped
2 garlic cloves, chopped
225g/8oz carrots
125g/4oz baby sweetcorn
125g/4oz green beans
125g/4oz courgettes (zucchini)
bunch of spring (green) onions
2tbsp lemon juice
1tsp toasted sesame oil
2 sachets ajitsuke nori
salt and freshly ground black pepper

Put the rice into a sieve, rinse well under cold running water, then put it into a saucepan together with the chopped fresh ginger, chopped garlic and 400ml/14fl oz/1¾ cups water. Bring to the boil, put the lid on the saucepan, turn the heat down low and leave to cook very gently for 45 minutes.

When the rice is cooked, leave it to stand, still covered, for a few minutes while you prepare the vegetables. Heat 1cm/½ in of water in a large saucepan and bring to the boil. While the water is coming to the boil, slice the carrots diagonally, halve the sweetcorn diagonally, cut the beans in half, slice the courgettes (zucchini) and chop the spring (green) onions. Add the carrots to the boiling water, then the sweetcorn, followed by the green beans, courgettes (zucchini) and spring (green) onions, in layers. The idea is to put the slowest-cooking vegetables at the bottom of the pan. Bring back to the boil, put the lid on the saucepan, and boil for about 4 minutes, or until the vegetables are tender but still crunchy — or cook them a little longer if you like them softer. Drain the vegtables in a colander, return them to the pan and toss well with the lemon juice, the sesame oil, ajitsuke nori or chopped fresh parsley and some salt and freshly ground black pepper. Serve immediately with the ginger rice.

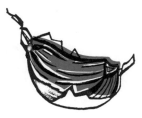

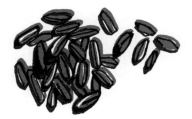

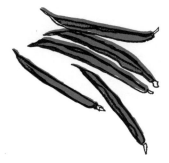

millet and onion pilaf with cumin and peas

Serve this with Yogurt and Fresh Herb Dressing (page 41) and a lightly cooked green vegetable, or a tomato salad.

serves 2

175g/6oz/scant 1 cup millet
350ml/12fl oz/1½ cups boiling water
1 onion, finely sliced
½ tsp cumin
1 tomato, chopped
125g/4oz/1 cup frozen peas
1tbsp freshly-squeezed lemon juice
salt and freshly ground black pepper

Put the millet into a saucepan, set over a moderate heat, and stir for 2–3 minutes, until the millet smells toasted and starts to jump around. Then, standing well back, add the boiling water. Cover the pan and leave off the heat for 1 hour, to soak.

Put the onion into a non-stick saucepan and cook, without any additional fat or liquid, for 6–7 minutes, until it is flecked with brown, stirring it often to prevent sticking. Add the cumin and stir over the heat for a few seconds until it smells aromatic. Stir in the tomato and the millet and its liquid. Bring to the boil, cover, reduce the heat, and leave to cook very gently for 35 minutes. Now add the peas, but don't stir them in. Cover and cook for a further 5 minutes. Remove from the heat and leave to stand for 10–15 minutes. Gently stir in the lemon juice and season with salt and freshly ground black pepper.

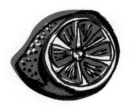

rice, red beans and vegetables

In this recipe, golden rice is flecked with red kidney beans and green, red and orange vegetables. Serve with a green salad.

serves 4

Put the onion into a non-stick saucepan and cook, without any additional fat or liquid, for 6–7 minutes, until it is flecked with brown, stirring it often to prevent sticking. Add the garlic and stir over the heat for a few seconds until it smells aromatic, then add the rice, turmeric, tomatoes, water and some salt. Bring to the boil, cover and simmer for 20 minutes. Add the carrot – don't stir in. Ten minutes later, add the rest of vegetables and beans; again, don't stir them in. Cook for further 10 minutes (40 minutes in all), then remove from heat and leave to stand for 15 minutes. Mix gently with a fork and add freshly ground black pepper and more salt if necessary.

2 onions, finely chopped
2 garlic cloves, crushed
350g/12oz/1¾ cups brown rice
1tbsp turmeric powder
4 tomatoes, peeled and chopped
850ml/30fl oz/3¾ cups water
salt and freshly ground black pepper
4 carrots, diced
2 courgettes (zucchini), sliced
1 sweet red pepper, deseeded and chopped
425g/15oz can red kidney beans, drained and rinsed

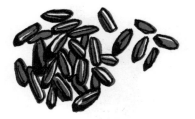

quinoa with sweet vegetables

Sweet vegetables are perfect for enhancing the slight bitterness of quinoa, as they do in this recipe. If there's any left over, it's also nice cold. It's important to rinse the quinoa thoroughly before cooking, as explained on page 63.

serves 4

2 carrots, finely diced
1 sweet red pepper, deseeded and diced
1 garlic clove, finely sliced
4 tomatoes, chopped
175g/6oz/scant 1 cup quinoa, washed and drained
400ml/14fl oz/1¾ cups vegetable stock or water
125g/4oz/ ⅔ cup sweetcorn, frozen or cut from the cob
salt and freshly ground black pepper

Put the carrot and sweet pepper into a non-stick saucepan and cook, without any additional fat or liquid, for 6–7 minutes, until they are flecked with brown, stirring often to prevent sticking. Add the garlic, tomatoes, drained quinoa and stock or water. Bring to the boil, cover, reduce the heat, and leave to cook very gently for 15 minutes.

Add the sweetcorn. Cover and cook for a further 5 minutes. Remove from the heat and leave to stand for 10–15 minutes, to make the grains dry and fluffy. Season with salt and freshly ground black pepper and gently stir through the rice.

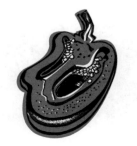

spiced vegetable rice

This is a lovely curry dish – spicy golden rice garnished with slices of tomato and chopped fresh coriander (cilantro). Serve it as it is, perhaps with a raita of cucumber mixed with plain yogurt, or Curry Sauce (page 136) goes well with it.

serves 4

Put the onion into a non-stick saucepan and cook, without any additional fat or liquid, for 6–7 minutes, until it is flecked with brown, stirring it often to prevent sticking. Add the garlic, bay leaf and spices and stir over the heat for a few seconds until they smell aromatic. Add the rice, okra, water and some salt. Bring to the boil, cover, turn the heat right down and leave to cook very gently for 40 minutes. Alternatively, it can be cooked in a preheated oven for 40 minutes at 200°C/400°F/gas mark 6.

Ten minutes before the rice is ready, add the peas – just tip them on top without stirring. When the rice is ready, remove the saucepan from the heat and leave it to stand, still covered, for 10 minutes. Then fork the rice through lightly and serve it garnished with some sliced tomato and the coriander (cilantro).

1 onion, chopped
1 large garlic clove, crushed
1 bay leaf
2tsp turmeric
4–5 cardamom pods
piece of cinnamon stick
pinch of ground cloves
275g/10oz/1½ cups brown rice
125g/4oz okra, trimmed if necessary
500ml/18fl oz/2¼ cups water
salt
125g/4oz/1 cup frozen peas

to serve
1 tomato, sliced
2tbsp chopped fresh coriander (cilantro)

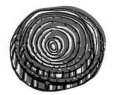

pasta

I've used wholewheat pasta in all of these recipes except for one, which uses buckwheat noodles. As I've said elsewhere, using wholegrain flours and products is, for many people, an integral part of low-sugar cooking because of the effect of refined 'white' products on blood sugar levels. Wholewheat pasta is widely available in a variety of different shapes; it's got a nutty flavour and is rather heavier than white pasta, but you soon get used to it. With a good flavoursome sauce or tasty ingredients added it can be very good.

If you can't eat wheat, then look for some of the alternative types of pasta now available: pasta made from corn, vegetables or millet, for instance. These are available from good health food stores. The ones that I've tried tasted good but it was very easy to over-cook them; I found they needed far less time than the packet said. So keep trying the pasta as it cooks and stop cooking immediately it is tender because with these non-wheat pastas there doesn't seem to be much leeway between perfectly al dente and hopelessly soggy.

rigatoni with tomato sauce

Tomato sauce on a chunky pasta like rigatoni makes a very satisfying dish.

serves 2

1 onion, chopped

1 large garlic clove, chopped

425g/15oz can tomatoes in juice

salt and freshly ground black pepper

6 basil leaves, torn

200g/7oz wholewheat rigatoni

Start by making the sauce. Put the onion into a non-stick pan, cover and cook gently for 6–7 minutes, until the onion is tender and lightly browned, stirring from time to time. Add the garlic and cook for a few seconds. Add the tomatoes, chopping them up a bit in the pan with the spoon. Bring to the boil and leave to boil gently, uncovered, for 10–15 minutes, until the mixture is thick. Season with salt and freshly ground black pepper.

While the sauce is cooking, bring a large panful of water to the boil for the pasta. Add the pasta and a good teaspoon of salt and stir. Let the pasta boil, uncovered, for 8–10 minutes, or until just tender.

Drain the pasta and either return it to the saucepan and mix with the sauce, or divide it between two plates and spoon the sauce on top. Either way, scatter with the torn basil leaves.

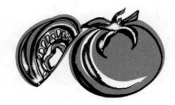

conchiglie with creamy broccoli sauce

In this recipe conchiglie is served with a creamy broccoli sauce flavoured with nutmeg and lemon juice. Ensure you have the sauce ready before beginning the recipe.

serves 2

Fill a large saucepan with 2 litres/70fl oz/9 cups of water and bring to the boil for the pasta. Add the pasta with a good teaspoon of salt and give the pasta a quick stir. Briefly put the lid on until it starts to lift, showing that the water has come back to the boil, then let the pasta bubble away, uncovered, for 8–10 minutes, or until it is tender but still has some bite to it.

Meanwhile, cook the broccoli in a little boiling water for 3–4 minutes, or until it is just tender, then drain and add to the béchamel sauce in a medium-sized saucepan. Heat the sauce through gently, adding salt, freshly ground black pepper, grated nutmeg and maybe a squeeze of lemon juice to taste.

Drain the pasta and either return it to the saucepan and mix with the sauce, or divide it between two plates and spoon the sauce on top.

200g/7oz wholewheat conchiglie
salt
225g/8oz/4 cups broccoli florets, roughly chopped
1 quantity of Béchamel Sauce, page 132
freshly ground black pepper
freshly grated nutmeg
squeeze of lemon juice, optional

macaroni and leek pie

This is a non-cheesy, non-dairy version of macaroni cheese, and despite being very low in fat, it tastes really creamy. It can be finished under the grill (broiler) or in the oven. Serve with a tomato salad.

serves 4

175g/6oz wholewheat macaroni
225g/8oz/2 cups sliced leeks
3 quantities of Onion Sauce, page 132
1tsp mustard powder
salt and freshly ground black pepper
4tbsp rolled oats and rice flakes mixed, or just rolled oats

Preheat the oven to 200°C/400°F/gas mark 6.

Bring a large saucepan of water to the boil, put in the pasta and cook, uncovered, for 8–10 minutes, or as directed on the packet, until the pasta is just tender, then drain. Meanwhile, cook the leeks in boiling water to cover until tender – about 10 minutes – and then drain.

Mix the pasta with the sauce, mustard powder, leeks and plenty of salt and freshly ground black pepper. Pour into a large shallow casserole dish and sprinkle the oats and rice flakes on top. Bake for 20–30 minutes, until the inside is hot and bubbling and the top golden brown and crisp.

variation

macaroni and asparagus pie

For this delicious variation, use 225g/8oz trimmed asparagus, cut into 2cm/1 in lengths and cooked until tender, instead of the leeks.

spaghetti with lentil bolognese

For a warming, comforting dish that's also easy to make, this dish is hard to beat.

serves 4

Put the onion, celery and carrot into a non-stick saucepan and cook, without any additional fat or liquid, for 6–7 minutes, until they are flecked with brown, stirring often to prevent sticking. Add the garlic and cook for a few seconds. Add the tomatoes, chopping them up a bit in the pan with the spoon. Drain the lentils, rinse in cold water and add to the pan. Bring to the boil, then turn the heat down and leave to boil gently, uncovered, for 10–15 minutes, until the mixture is thick. Season with salt and freshly ground black pepper.

Meanwhile, cook the pasta. Fill a large saucepan with 2 litres/70fl oz/9 cups of water and bring to the boil. Add a good teaspoonful of salt and the spaghetti, holding it straight up and bending it into the water as it softens. Give it a quick stir, briefly put the lid on until it starts to lift, showing that the water has come back to the boil, then let the pasta bubble away, uncovered, for 8–10 minutes, or until it is tender but still has some bite to it.

Drain the spaghetti by tipping it all into a colander placed in the sink, then divide it between serving plates and spoon the bolognese sauce on top.

1 onion, chopped
1 celery stalk, finely chopped
1 carrot, finely diced
1 large garlic clove, chopped
425g/15oz can tomatoes in juice
425g/15oz can green lentils
salt and freshly ground black pepper
200g/7oz wholewheat spaghetti

spaghetti with tomato and caper sauce

Look for capers preserved in salt, not vinegar; they can be bought from good food shops and may be found in the special selections at some large supermarkets.

serves 2

1 onion, chopped

1 large garlic clove, chopped

425g/15oz can tomatoes in juice

1tbsp capers, rinsed and drained

salt and freshly ground black pepper

200g/7oz wholewheat spaghetti

Start by making the sauce. Put the onion into a non-stick saucepan and cook, without any additional fat or liquid, for 6–7 minutes, until it is flecked with brown, stirring it often to prevent sticking. Add the garlic, cook for a few seconds, then add the tomatoes, chopping them up a bit in the pan with the spoon. Add the capers, then bring to the boil and leave to boil gently, uncovered, for 10–15 minutes, until the mixture is thick. Season with salt and freshly ground black pepper.

Meanwhile, cook the pasta. Fill a large saucepan with 2 litres/70fl oz/9 cups of water and bring to the boil. Add a good teaspoonful of salt and the spaghetti, holding it straight up and bending it into the water as it softens. Give it a quick stir, briefly put the lid on until it starts to lift, showing that the water has come back to the boil, then let the pasta bubble away, uncovered, for 8–10 minutes, or until it is tender but still has some bite to it.

Drain the pasta and either return it to the saucepan and mix with the sauce, or divide it between two plates and spoon the sauce on top.

fettuccine with herb sauce

This is a very herby sauce which is delicious with fettuccine. You could use other mixtures of herbs if you prefer.

serves 2

Fill a large saucepan with 2 litres/70fl oz/9 cups of water and bring to the boil for the pasta. Add the pasta with a good teaspoonful of salt and give the pasta a quick stir. Briefly put the lid on until it starts to lift, showing that the water has come back to the boil, then let the pasta bubble away, uncovered, for 8–10 minutes, or until it is tender but still has some bite to it.

When the pasta is almost ready, heat the sauce through gently, adding the fresh herbs and salt, freshly ground black pepper, grated nutmeg and maybe a squeeze of lemon juice to taste.

Drain the pasta and either return it to the saucepan and mix with the sauce, or divide it between two plates and spoon the sauce on top.

200g/7oz wholewheat fettuccine
salt
1 quantity of Béchamel Sauce or Onion Sauce, page 132
1tbsp chopped fresh parsley
1tbsp chopped fresh chives
1tbsp chopped fresh tarragon
freshly ground black pepper
freshly grated nutmeg
squeeze of lemon juice, optional

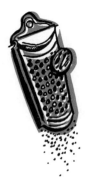

fusilli with creamy leek sauce

Shred the leeks finely for this recipe so that they can be distributed throughout the creamy sauce.

serves 2

200g/7oz wholewheat fusilli
salt
225g/8oz/2 cups finely sliced leeks
1 quantity of Béchamel Sauce, page 132
freshly ground black pepper
freshly grated nutmeg
squeeze of lemon juice, optional
1tbsp chopped fresh parsley, to serve

Fill a large saucepan with 2 litres/70fl oz/9 cups of water and bring to the boil for the pasta. Add the pasta with a good teaspoonful of salt and give the pasta a quick stir. Briefly put the lid on until it starts to lift, showing that the water has come back to the boil, then let the pasta bubble away, uncovered, for 8–10 minutes, or until it is tender but still has some bite to it.

Meanwhile, cover the leeks in boiling water and cook for 5–6 minutes, or until tender, then drain and add to the béchamel sauce in a medium-sized saucepan. Heat the sauce through gently, adding salt, freshly ground black pepper, grated nutmeg and maybe a squeeze of lemon juice to taste.

Drain the pasta and either return it to the saucepan and mix with the sauce, or divide it between two plates and spoon the sauce on top. Sprinkle with the chopped parsley and serve.

buckwheat noodles and oriental vegetables

This is good flavoured with soy sauce if your diet allows this; if not, use a good squeeze of lemon juice.

serves 4

Fill a large saucepan with 2 litres/70fl oz/9 cups of water and bring to the boil. Add the buckwheat noodles and a couple of teaspoons of salt. Give it a quick stir, briefly put the lid on until it starts to lift, showing that the water has come back to the boil, then let the noodles bubble away, uncovered, for 5 minutes, or as directed on the packet.

Meanwhile, prepare the vegetables. Heat the oil in a medium-sized saucepan and add the garlic and ginger. Stir for 30 seconds, then add the spring (green) onions, mangetout (snowpeas) and sweetcorn and stir-fry for 2–3 minutes until all the vegetables are hot.

Drain the noodles by tipping them into a colander placed in the sink, then put them back into the still-warm pan, add the vegetable mixture, the soy sauce or lemon juice, the coriander (cilantro) and freshly ground black pepper, and toss gently. Check the seasoning and serve.

400g/14oz buckwheat
noodles
salt
1tsp olive oil
2 garlic cloves, crushed
1tsp grated fresh ginger
6 spring (green) onions,
chopped
125g/4oz mangetout
(snowpeas), sliced
diagonally
125g/4oz baby sweetcorn,
sliced diagonally
2tbsp soy sauce or lemon
juice
freshly ground black pepper
2–3tbsp chopped fresh
coriander (cilantro)

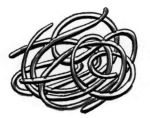

Making burgers and rissoles without fat might seem like a thankless task, but this turned out to be one of my favourite sections of this book. I found that the burgers or rissoles could be baked in the oven, cooked under the grill (broiler) or dry-fried in a non-stick frying pan. All these methods were successful, though my own preference is for the oven because it's the easiest; simply put them onto a baking tray, bake for 15–20 minutes then turn them and cook the other side.

One of the keys to success lies in non-stick equipment: a non-stick baking tray or baking tray lined with non-stick fabric or paper, if you're using the oven; a non-stick frying pan or grill (broiler) pan or baking tray if the dish is going under the grill (broiler). Having got the right equipment, the next important point is to make sure the mixture is moist enough; obviously it has to hold together, but make sure it's not too dry as there's no oil or butter to moisten it as it cooks. For coating the burgers, I suggest brown rice flour or polenta, which both give a lovely crisp finish.

burgers and rissoles

butter bean and sage patties

These patties are delicious served with creamy Butternut Squash and Garlic Sauce (page 135).

serves 4

1 onion, finely chopped
425g/15oz can butter or lima beans
1tbsp freshly-squeezed lemon juice
grated rind of ½ a lemon
2–3 fresh sage leaves, chopped
salt and freshly ground black pepper
2–3tbsp brown rice flour for coating

Preheat the oven to 200°C/400°F/gas mark 6.

Put the onion into a non-stick saucepan and cook, without any additional fat or liquid, for 6–7 minutes, until it is flecked with brown, stirring it often to prevent sticking. Drain the butter or lima beans, rinse under cold water, then add to the onion along with the lemon juice and rind and the sage. Mash well, to produce a mixture which holds together, making it as smooth or chunky as you like.

Spread the rice flour out on a flat plate or board. Divide the tofu mixture into 8 equal pieces, place on the rice flour and form into flat burgers, pressing them together well and making sure they're coated all over with the rice flour. Put them on a non-stick baking tray and bake for 20–30 minutes, turning them over after about 15 minutes, to cook both sides.

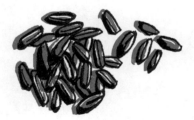

lentil burgers

These are good served in baps, normal burger-style, or with chutney and cooked vegetables or salad.

makes 8

Put the lentils in a saucepan with the water. Bring to the boil, then cover and leave to cook very gently for 20–25 minutes, or until the lentils are soft and pale and all the water has been absorbed. Cover the potatoes with water and boil until just tender, then drain and mash.

Preheat the oven to 200°C/400°F/Gas Mark 6.

Put the onion into a non-stick saucepan and cook, without any additional fat or liquid, for 6–7 minutes, until it is flecked with brown, stirring it often to prevent sticking. Add the lentils, mashed potato, thyme, oregano, grated nutmeg, parsley and salt and freshly ground black pepper.

Spread the rice flour out on a flat plate or board. Divide the lentil mixture into 8 equal pieces, place on the rice flour and form into flat burgers, pressing them together well and making sure they're coated all over with the rice flour. Put them on a non-stick baking tray and bake for 20–30 minutes, turning them over after about 15 minutes, to cook both sides.

175g/6oz/scant 1 cup split red lentils
200ml/7fl oz/¾ cup water
225g/8oz potatoes, peeled and cut into even-sized pieces
1 onion, chopped
½ tsp thyme
½ tsp oregano
freshly grated nutmeg
1tbsp chopped fresh parsley
salt and freshly ground black pepper
6–8tbsp brown rice flour for coating

polenta rounds with roasted peppers and basil

These are stunning to look at – rounds of golden polenta grilled (broiled) and topped with sweet red peppers and basil. Instant polenta is widely available, but if you want to be sure of a GMO- and additive-free product, I think it's probably safer to use the traditional type.

serves 4

175g/6oz/ heaping 1 cup polenta
1tsp salt
600ml/20fl oz/2½ cups water
2 large sweet red peppers
4 sprigs of basil

Put the polenta into a saucepan – non-stick helps, if you have one – with the salt. Add the water, a little at a time, stirring, to make a smooth mixture. Bring to the boil, stirring as it thickens, then turn the heat right down and leave to cook very gently, uncovered, for 20 minutes. A heat diffuser over the hot plate or flame is useful to avoid over-heating.

Spread the mixture into four 20cm/4 in circles using small plates or free-forming them on a baking tray or something similar, then leave them to go cold and firm.

Meanwhile, prepare the sweet peppers. Cut them in half, remove the core and seeds and put the halves, rounded-side up, on a baking tray or grill (broiler) pan. Cook under a hot grill (broiler) for 10–15 minutes, or until the peppers are tender and the skin blackened in places. When they have cooled a little, you can remove the papery skins if you wish, or leave them on – I prefer them on. Cut the peppers into strips.

Heat the grill (broiler). Transfer the polenta rounds to a grill (broiler) pan or baking tray that will fit under the grill (broiler) and cook for 15–20 minutes, until the tops

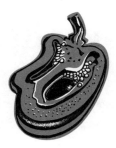

are crisp and browned in places, then turn them over and grill (broil) the other side for about 10 minutes, until crisp.

Place some pepper strips on each polenta round and top with the basil leaves.

variations

polenta rounds with asparagus

Make the polenta rounds as described above. Boil 225g/8oz tender trimmed asparagus spears in water until tender, or place under a grill (broiler) until tender and browned in places – about 10 minutes. Pile the asparagus spears on top of the grilled (broiled) polenta rounds.

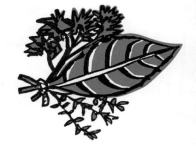

polenta rounds with tomato sauce and capers

Make and cook the polenta rounds as described above. Prepare a batch of Tomato Sauce (page 133), spread some on top of each grilled (broiled) polenta round, leaving the edges clear. Sprinkle with a few capers (the kind preserved in salt, rinsed before using) and serve.

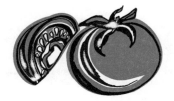

spicy bean burgers

These bean burgers are very low in fat yet full of flavour. Try them topped with a spoonful of Tomato Sauce (page 133).

makes 4

1 onion, finely chopped
1 small carrot, grated
½ sweet red pepper, deseeded and chopped
1 garlic clove, crushed
½ tsp ground coriander
425g/15oz can red kidney beans
salt and freshly ground black pepper
2–3tbsp brown rice flour for coating

Preheat the oven to 200°C/400°F/gas mark 6.

Put the onion, carrot and sweet pepper into a non-stick saucepan and cook, without any additional fat or liquid, for 6–7 minutes, until they are flecked with brown, stirring often to prevent sticking. Stir in the garlic and coriander and cook for a further minute, then remove from the heat. Mash the beans and add to the vegetable mixture with some salt and freshly ground black pepper.

Spread the rice flour out on a flat plate or board. Divide the red bean mixture into 4 equal pieces, place on the rice flour and form into flat burgers, pressing them together well and making sure they're coated all over with the rice flour. Put them on a non-stick baking tray and bake for 20–30 minutes, turning them over after about 15 minutes, to cook both sides. Serve hot or warm.

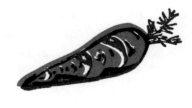

felafel with tsatsiki

This is a fat-free version of the popular Middle Eastern chick pea (garbanzo bean) patties, served with salad and tsatsiki.

makes 4

Preheat the oven to 200°C/400°F/gas mark 6.

Drain the chick peas (garbanzo beans) and rinse under cold water. Mash the chick peas (garbanzo beans) with all the remaining felafel ingredients, except for the brown rice flour.

Spread the rice flour out on a flat plate or board. Divide the chick pea (garbanzo bean) mixture into 4 equal pieces, place on the rice flour and form into flat burgers, pressing them together well and making sure they're coated all over with the rice flour. Put them onto a non-stick baking tray and bake for 20–30 minutes, turning them over after about 15 minutes, to cook both sides. Serve hot, or warm, on a bed of lettuce, surrounded by the tomato and cucumber and accompanied by the tsatsiki.

425g/15oz can chick peas (garbanzo beans)
25g/1oz/2tbsp very finely chopped onion
2tbsp chopped fresh parsley
1 garlic clove, crushed
1tsp ground coriander
salt and freshly ground black pepper
2–3tbsp brown rice flour for coating

to serve
crisp lettuce leaves
sliced tomatoes and cucumber
tsatsiki, page 17

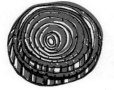

curried vegetable and tofu burgers with yogurt sauce

If you've wondered how to make tofu really tasty, try these. They're excellent with a yogurt and coriander (cilantro) sauce and some salad, cooked green beans or broccoli. If you've got a food processor, the vegetables can be cut into rough chunks then quickly chopped all together by pulsing in the food processor.

makes 8

1 onion, finely chopped
2 carrots, finely chopped
2 celery stalks, chopped
1 sweet red pepper, deseeded and chopped
2 garlic cloves, crushed
4–6tsp curry powder
285g/10oz packet tofu
salt and freshly ground black pepper
6–8tbsp brown rice flour for coating

for the sauce
150ml/5fl oz/⅔ cup low-fat plain yogurt
1tbsp freshly-squeezed lemon juice
1tbsp chopped fresh coriander (cilantro)
salt and freshly ground black pepper

Preheat the oven to 200°C/400°F/gas mark 6.

Put the onion, carrot, celery and sweet pepper into a non-stick saucepan and cook, without any additional fat or liquid, for 5 minutes so that they soften a little but are still very crunchy. Add the garlic and curry powder and cook for a further minute. Remove from the heat. Drain the tofu and whiz in the food processor, or mash very well, so that it is smooth-crumbly, like fine cottage cheese. Add this to the curry mixture and season with salt and freshly ground black pepper.

Spread the rice flour out on a flat plate or board. Divide the tofu mixture into 8 equal pieces, place on the rice flour and form into flat burgers, pressing them together well and making sure they're coated all over with the rice flour. Put them on a non-stick baking tray and bake for 20–30 minutes, turning them over after about 15 minutes, to cook both sides.

While the burgers are cooking, make the sauce by mixing all the ingredients together. Serve the sauce in a jug, with the burgers.

savoury bakes

This section contains a medley of dishes which need to be baked in the oven or under the grill (broiler); they include gratins, non-pastry pies (including a particularly good cottage pie), a red bean moussaka and a spiced lentil dish. In addition, there are a number of quiches and a pizza.

When I started experimenting with low-fat mixtures for these, I was surprised what successful results I got using ingredients such as potatoes, puréed beans, and even a tofu mix. Once they have been baked, the results are surprisingly not unlike pastry and these mixtures offer interesting possibilities for flavouring in a way that pastry doesn't. They are good both hot and cold, with a salad or cooked vegetables.

potato quiche with leek filling

A mashed potato mixture forms the shell of this quiche, while leeks in a creamy sauce provide the filling.

serves 4–6

450g/1lb potatoes, peeled and cut into even-sized pieces

salt and freshly ground black pepper

for the filling

2 good tbsp brown rice flour

300ml/10fl oz/1¼ cups soya milk

225g/8oz/2 cups thinly-sliced leek

2tbsp chopped fresh parsley

salt and freshly ground black pepper

freshly grated nutmeg

Preheat the oven to 200°C/400°F/gas mark 6.

To make the base, first cover the potatoes in water and boil until tender. Drain and mash with some salt and freshly ground black pepper. The mixture needs to be quite dry. Spoon the mixture into an 18–20cm/7½–8 in fairly shallow flan dish, spreading it evenly and extending it up the sides to create a flan case. Bake for about 15 minutes, until set and lightly browned.

While the potatoes are cooking, make the sauce. Put the rice flour into a saucepan and add the soya milk gradually, stirring, to make a smooth mixture. Add the leek and stir over the heat until the mixture thickens. Turn the heat down very low (use a heat diffuser if you have one), cover and leave to cook very gently for 10 minutes, until the leek is tender, stirring from time to time. Stir in the parsley and season with salt and freshly ground black pepper.

Spoon the leek mixture into the potato flan, grate some nutmeg over the top and serve immediately, or return to the oven for 10–15 minutes to heat through before serving.

bean quiche with onion filling

Mashed beans make a surprisingly good base for a quiche. Here the filling is made from onions in a creamy sauce, but other vegetables, such as leeks, broccoli, courgettes (zucchini), or strips of grilled (broiled) sweet red pepper, are also good.

serves 4–6

Preheat the oven to 200°C/400°F/gas mark 6.

To make the base, drain and rinse the beans, drain again then mash thoroughly by hand or in a food processor or blender. Spoon the mixture into an 18–20cm/7½–8 in fairly shallow flan dish, spreading it evenly and extending it up the sides to create a flan case. Bake for about 15 minutes, until set and lightly browned.

While the flan is cooking, make the filling. Put the rice flour into a saucepan and add the soya milk gradually, stirring, to make a smooth mixture. Add the chopped onion and the bay leaf, then stir over the heat until the mixture thickens. Turn the heat down very low (use a heat diffuser if you have one), cover and leave to cook very gently for 10 minutes, until the onion is tender, stirring from time to time. Remove the bay leaf and season the mixture with salt, freshly ground black pepper and freshly grated nutmeg.

Spoon the onion mixture into the bean flan, arrange the tomato slices over the top then put it back into the oven for 5–10 minutes more, to cook the tomato slices and make it piping hot.

425g/15oz cannellini, butter or lima beans
salt and freshly ground black pepper

for the filling
2 good tbsp brown rice flour
300ml/10fl oz/1¼ cups soya milk
1 onion, finely chopped
1 bay leaf
salt and freshly ground black pepper
freshly grated nutmeg
1 tomato, finely sliced

curried tofu quiche with baby corn filling

This recipe reverses the usual role for tofu in quiches: here it's used to make the deliciously spicy crust, rather than the filling.

serves 6

1 onion, finely chopped

2 carrots, finely chopped

2 celery stalks, chopped

1 sweet red pepper, deseeded and chopped

2 garlic cloves, crushed

4–6tsp mild or medium curry powder

285g/10oz packet tofu, drained

salt and freshly ground black pepper

for the filling

125g/4oz baby sweetcorn

Preheat the oven to 200°C/400°F/gas mark 6.

Put the onion, carrot, celery and sweet pepper into a non-stick saucepan and cook, without any additional fat or liquid, for 5 minutes, so that they soften a little but are still very crunchy. Add the garlic and curry powder and cook for a further minute. Remove from the heat. Whiz the tofu in the food processor, or mash very well, so that it is smooth-crumbly, like fine cottage cheese. Add the tofu to the curry mixture and season with salt and freshly ground black pepper.

Spoon the mixture into an 18–20cm/7½–8 in fairly shallow flan dish, spreading it evenly and extending it up the sides to create a flan case. Bake for about 15 minutes, until set and lightly browned.

Meanwhile, cook the baby sweetcorn in boiling water for 4–5 minutes until tender; drain. Arrange the baby sweetcorn in the flan, close together, radiating from the centre like the spokes of a wheel. Serve immediately.

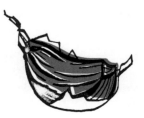

potato pizza

This is best made in a fairly large non-stick frying pan. If the mixture is stiff enough, it will be possible to turn the pizza over with a fish slice, but if you have difficulty with this, invert a large dinner plate over the frying pan, turn the pizza out on to this, then slide it back into the frying pan. The pizza is finished under the grill (broiler); some cheese could be added at this point for anyone who isn't eating low fat.

serves 2

To make the base, first cover the potatoes in water and boil until tender. Drain and mash with some salt and freshly ground black pepper. The mixture needs to be quite dry but add a little soya milk if necessary, to make it hold together.

While the potatoes are cooking, prepare the topping. Heat the oil in a medium-sized saucepan, add the onion and fry gently, covered, for 10 minutes, stirring from time to time to prevent sticking. Add the garlic, cook for a few seconds, then add the tomatoes, chopping them up a bit in the pan with the spoon. Bring to the boil, then leave to boil gently, uncovered, for 10–15 minutes, until the mixture is thick. Season with salt and freshly ground black pepper.

Sprinkle the rice flour on a board, turn the potato on to this and form into a flat circle which will fit your frying pan, preferably a non-stick one. Heat the frying pan, add the potato and press down to fill the pan. Cook for 4–5 minutes, until browned on the base, then turn it over with a fish slice and cook the other side. Heat the grill (broiler). Spread the tomato sauce over the pizza and arrange the tomato slices on top. Put the frying pan under the grill (broiler) for about 5 minutes, until the tomatoes have softened and browned slightly.

450g/1lb potatoes, peeled and cut into even-sized pieces
salt and freshly ground black pepper
a few drops soya milk, optional
1–2tbsp brown rice flour

for the topping
1tsp olive oil
1 onion, chopped
1 large garlic clove, chopped
425g/15oz can tomatoes in juice
2 tomatoes, sliced
½ tsp dried oregano

chestnut and sage loaf

This is a moist savoury loaf which is good either hot or cold. Serve with some Brown Onion Sauce (page 138) and some lightly-cooked savoy cabbage or Brussels sprouts.

serves 6

1 large onion, chopped
2 celery stalks, finely chopped
2 garlic cloves, crushed
2tbsp chopped fresh sage or 1tsp dried sage
2 x 240g/8oz cans peeled chestnuts
1tbsp freshly-squeezed lemon juice
2 egg whites
salt and freshly ground black pepper
1 sage leaf, to garnish

Preheat the oven to 180°C/350°F/gas mark 4.

Prepare a 450g/1lb loaf pan by lining the base and narrow sides with a long strip of silicon paper.

Put the onion, celery and garlic into a non-stick saucepan and cook, without any additional fat or liquid, for 6–7 minutes, until they are flecked with brown, stirring often to prevent sticking. Mash the chestnuts and add to the onion mixture along with the sage, lemon juice and egg whites. Season with salt and freshly ground black pepper.

Lay the sage leaf in the base of the prepared loaf pan and spoon the chestnut mixture on top. Smooth over the surface and cover with a piece of foil. Bake the loaf for 1 hour. To serve, slip a knife around the sides of the loaf and turn out on to a warm dish.

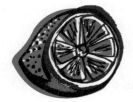

classic lentil roast

This is lovely in thick slices with Fat-free Garlicky Roast Potatoes (page 111) and Brussels Sprouts with Ginger (page 123). It's also good cold, with Yogurt and Fresh Herb Dressing (page 41) and a salad.

serves 4

Preheat the oven to 200°C/400°F/gas mark 6.

Put the lentils into a saucepan with the water, bring to the boil, then turn the heat down and cook over a gentle heat for 20 minutes, or until the lentils are beigy-gold and soft, and all the water has disappeared. They will be very dry.

While the lentils are cooking, put the onion into a non-stick saucepan and cook, without any additional fat or liquid, for 6–7 minutes, until they are flecked with brown and getting soft, stirring often to prevent sticking. Add the garlic and cook for a minute or two longer. Mix the onions with the lentils, lemon juice and rind, and plenty of salt and freshly ground black pepper. The mixture will be dry enough to hold together; use your hands to form it into a roll shape and place on a non-stick baking tray, or a baking tray lined with a piece of non-stick baking parchment. Bake for about 45 minutes, until crisp on the outside.

500g/1lb 2oz/2½ cups split red lentils
1 litre/35fl oz/4½ cups water
4 large onions, chopped
2 garlic cloves, crushed
grated rind and juice of 1 lemon
salt and freshly ground black pepper

red bean moussaka

Delicious though it is, moussaka is usually quite high in fat even when made with beans instead of meat. This recipe manages to remove the fat whilst retaining the flavour. For a slightly more lenient version, you could spray the aubergine (eggplant) slices with a little home-made oil and water spray, *see page xv.*

serves 6

1 large onion, chopped

2 aubergines (eggplants), sliced into 6mm/¼ in circles

425g/15oz can red kidney beans

425g/15oz can tomatoes in juice

½ tsp cinnamon

salt and freshly ground black pepper

2 quantities Béchamel Sauce, page 132

Preheat the oven to 180°C/350°F/gas mark 4.

Put the onion into a non-stick saucepan and cook, without any additional fat or liquid, for 6–7 minutes, until it is flecked with brown, stirring it often to prevent sticking. Meanwhile, brush the aubergine (eggplant) slices on both sides with water, place in a shallow container, cover with a plate and microwave on high for about 8 minutes, or until tender; or cook them in a little boiling water for 5–6 minutes, until tender. Drain well.

Drain the beans and rinse under cold water. Add the beans to the onion, along with the tomatoes, mashing them both with the spoon, then add the cinnamon and season with salt and freshly ground black pepper.

Place half the aubergine (eggplant) slices in the base of a shallow ovenproof dish, cover with half the red bean mixture and then half the sauce. Repeat the layers, ending with the sauce, then bake for 1 hour.

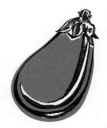

vegetable and lentil gratin

This gratin can be baked as soon as you've assembled it or it can be prepared in advance ready for baking later – either way it's a good winter dish.

serves 4

Put the onion into a non-stick saucepan and cook, without any additional fat or liquid, for 6-7 minutes, until it is flecked with brown, stirring it often to prevent sticking. Add the carrot and celery, stir, then cover and cook over a gentle heat for a further 10 minutes, until all the vegetables are softening. Keep an eye on them and stir often to prevent sticking.

Put the lentils into a sieve and wash them quickly under cold water, then add them to the saucepan and stir to distribute all the ingredients. Add the water and season with salt and freshly ground black pepper. Bring to the boil, cover and turn the heat down so that the mixture just simmers. Leave to cook for 25–30 minutes, until the vegetables are tender and the lentils soft and pale.

Transfer the lentil and vegetable mixture to a shallow dish that will fit under the grill (broiler) and sprinkle the oat flakes, or oat and rice flakes, on top. Place under a hot grill (broiler) for 10–15 minutes, or until the topping is golden brown and crisp. If you are preparing the gratin in advance, add the topping at the last minute and bake in a preheated 180°C/350°F/gas mark 4 oven for 30–40 minutes, until the mixture is heated through and the topping golden and crisp.

2 onions, chopped
2 large carrots, cut into 5mm/¼ in dice
2 large celery stalks, cut into 5mm/¼ in dice
225g/8oz/heaping 1 cup red lentils
600ml/20fl oz/2½ cups water
salt and freshly ground black pepper
3–4 good tbsp rolled oats or a mixture of oats and rice flakes

spiced lentils

This is a simple casserole of lentils baked with garlic and coriander. It goes well with Root Vegetables in Turmeric Sauce (page 57).

serves 4–6

2 large onions, finely chopped
4 large garlic cloves, crushed
4tsp ground coriander
2 x 425g/15oz cans green lentils
300ml/10fl oz/1¼ cups water
salt and freshly ground black pepper

Preheat the oven to 160°C/325°F/gas mark 3.

Put the onion into a non-stick saucepan and cook, without any additional fat or liquid, for 6–7 minutes, until it is flecked with brown, stirring it often to prevent sticking. Stir in the garlic and coriander. Cook over the heat for a few seconds until they smell aromatic. Drain the lentils and rinse under cold water, then add to the onion mixture and stir them around so that they all get coated with the onion and spices. Add the water and bring to the boil. Transfer to a casserole dish, cover and bake for 40–60 minutes, until the lentils are tender and have absorbed the water. Season with salt and freshly ground black pepper.

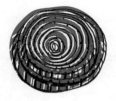

butter bean cottage pie with thyme mash

Serve this delicious pie with a cooked green vegetable.

serves 4

Put the onion into a non-stick saucepan and cook, without any additional fat or liquid, for 6–7 minutes, until it is flecked with brown, stirring it often to prevent sticking. Add the celery, leek, parsnip, carrot and garlic and stir. Cover and cook over a gentle heat for 10 minutes, until all the vegetables are softening. Keep an eye on them and stir often to prevent sticking. Drain the butter or lima beans and rinse in a sieve under cold water. Add to the pan, along with the sweetcorn, tomatoes and tomato juice. Mash the tomatoes with the spoon to break them up a bit. Bring to the boil, cover, turn down the heat and leave to simmer for a further 20–30 minutes, until all the vegetables are tender. Season with salt and freshly ground black pepper.

Meanwhile, boil the potatoes until tender. Drain and mash with enough soya milk to produce a creamy consistency, add the thyme and season with salt and freshly ground pepper.

Preheat the grill (broiler). If necessary, transfer the vegetable mixture to a casserole dish which will fit under the grill (broiler), then spread the potato on top. Make ridges on top with a fork. Grill (broil) for about 10 minutes, until browned on top.

2 onions, chopped
2 celery stalks, sliced
4 leeks, sliced
1 large parsnip, peeled and sliced
225g/8oz carrots, diced
2–3 garlic cloves, chopped
425g/15oz can butter or lima beans
325g/11oz can sweetcorn, drained
425g/15oz can tomatoes in juice
300ml/10fl oz/1¼ cups tomato juice
salt and freshly ground black pepper

for the topping
450g/1lb potatoes, peeled and cut into even-sized pieces
a little soya milk
1tbsp chopped fresh thyme
salt and freshly ground black pepper

quick bean
and sweetcorn pie

A mixture which children enjoy. Use no-sugar, no-salt baked beans which you can buy at
health shops and large supermarkets.

serves 4

750g/1½ lb potatoes,
peeled and cut into
even-sized pieces
a little soya milk
salt and freshly ground
black pepper
425g/15oz can no-salt,
no-sugar baked beans
350g/12oz can no-salt, no-
sugar sweetcorn, drained

Cover the potatoes with water and boil until tender, then
drain and mash with enough soya milk to make a creamy
consistency. Season with salt and freshly ground black
pepper. Put the baked beans and sweetcorn into a
saucepan and heat.

Preheat the grill (broiler). Spread half the potato into
a casserole dish which will fit under your grill (broiler)
and pour the beans and sweetcorn over the top. Spoon the
remaining potato over the beans, spread it to the edges
and make ridges on top with a fork. Grill (broil) for about
10 minutes, until browned on top.

sweet red pepper
and chestnut casserole

This hearty winter casserole is excellent served with a baked potato. Some lightly-cooked cabbage or sprouts go very well with it, too, providing a classic combination of flavours.

serves 4

Put the onion, sweet pepper and celery into a non-stick saucepan and cook, without any additional fat or liquid, for 6–7 minutes, until they are flecked with brown and getting soft, stirring often to prevent sticking. Add the tomatoes, breaking them up with the spoon once they're in the pan, the chestnuts and stock or water. Bring to the boil, reduce the heat, cover and leave to boil gently for 30 minutes, stirring occasionally, until the vegetables are very tender. Season with salt and freshly ground black pepper.

2 onions, chopped
2 sweet red peppers, deseeded and chopped
1 head celery, finely sliced
425g/15oz can tomatoes in juice
2 cans whole chestnuts
400ml/14fl oz/1¾ cups vegetable stock or water
salt and freshly ground black pepper

variation

sweet red pepper and bean casserole

For a delicious variation, try this recipe using the drained contents of two 425g/15oz cans of beans – butter, lima beans or chick peas (garbanzo beans) are particularly good – instead of the chestnuts.

vegetable pie

This is very simple, yet tasty. Serve with a cooked green vegetable such as broccoli or fresh peas.

serves 4

450g/1lb potatoes cut into
3mm/⅛ in slices
2 onions, thinly sliced
425g/15oz can chopped
tomatoes in juice
salt and freshly ground
black pepper
1tsp dried oregano
1 quantity Béchamel Sauce,
page 132

Preheat the oven to 180°C/350°F/gas mark 4.

Cook the potato slices in boiling water until tender — about 10 minutes; drain. Mix together the potato slices, onion, tomato and oregano and season with salt and freshly ground black pepper. Spoon the mixture into a shallow dish and pour the béchamel sauce over the top. Bake for about 45 minutes, until lightly browned.

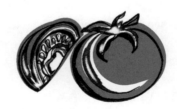

sweetcorn and courgette bake

This is another quick bake which is popular with children; it's good with Tomato Sauce (page 133).

serves 3–4

Preheat the oven to 200°C/400°F/gas mark 6.

Cook the courgettes (zucchini) in 1cm/½ in fast-boiling water for about 4 minutes, or until tender. Drain and put into a bowl with the sweetcorn, onion sauce and egg white. Mix together and season with some salt and freshly ground black pepper. Spoon the mixture into a shallow ovenproof dish and bake for 30–40 minutes.

225g/8oz courgettes (zucchini), sliced
340g/12oz can sweetcorn
1 quantity of Onion Sauce, page 132
1 egg white
salt and freshly ground black pepper

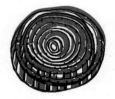

vegetables

You really don't need lots of oil, cream and butter to make vegetables taste good. Cooked carefully and flavoured with fresh herbs, spices, garlic, fresh ginger and lemon or lime juice, low-fat vegetable dishes can be exciting and delicious.

The majority of recipes in this section contain no oil or butter, although there are one or two exceptions. I couldn't resist putting in low-fat (as well as fat-free) versions of chips and roast potatoes, and wanted to include grilled Mediterranean vegetables but I haven't found a way of making that completely fat-free. However, you will find an excellent fat-free ratatouille in this section along with Fat-free Fried Onions, Brussels Sprouts with Ginger and, one of my special favourites, beautifully spicy Cauliflower with Turmeric and Cumin.

low-fat chips

These chips (French fries) are made with just a little oil: 5 grams of fat for the full portion.

serves 1

350g/12oz potato
1tsp olive oil

Preheat the oven to 200°C/400°F/gas mark 6.
   Cut the potato into flat chunky chips (French fries) – about 5cm/2 in long and 2cm/¾-in wide. Place the cut potatoes in a bowl, sprinkle with the oil and toss them together with your hands. Place the chips (French fries) on a non-stick baking tray (or a baking tray covered with non-stick parchment or material) and bake for about 25 minutes, or until they're crisp and golden. I find there's no need to turn them during the cooking, but you do need to eat them quickly while they're really crisp.

fat-free chips

This is the strictest recipe for chips (French fries) — they're made without a drop of oil, yet are surprisingly crisp and tasty to eat.

serves 1

350g/12oz potato

Preheat the oven to 200°C/400°F/gas mark 6.
   Part-cook the potato by pricking it with a fork and microwaving on full power for 4 minutes, until it's a bit soft around the edges but still raw in the middle. Cut the potato into flat chunky chips – about 5cm/2 in long and 2cm/¾ in wide. Place the chips (French fries) on a non-stick baking tray (or a baking tray covered with non-stick parchment or material) and bake for about 25 minutes, or until they're crisp and golden. I find there's no need to turn them during the cooking, but you do need to eat them quickly while they're really crisp.

fat-free fried onions

These onions are tender, full of flavour and delicious.

serves 4

Put the onion into a non-stick pan, cover and cook gently
for about 7 minutes, until the onion is tender and lightly
browned, stirring from time to time. Add half of the stock
or water, bring to the boil and let it bubble away until
almost all the liquid has disappeared, then pour in the
remaining stock or water and repeat the process until you
have tender, glossy brown onions in just a little syrupy
liquid. Season with salt and freshly ground black pepper
and serve.

6 onions, finely sliced
400ml/14fl oz/1¾ cups
vegetable stock or water
salt and freshly ground
black pepper

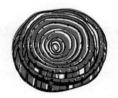

low-fat roast potatoes

You'll be surprised how good these low-fat potatoes taste.

serves 4

500g/1lb 2oz small–
medium potatoes, peeled
and halved
1tsp olive oil

Preheat the oven to 230°C/450°F/gas mark 8.

Parboil the potatoes for 6–7 minutes, until they are becoming tender but are not at all soggy. Drain, put into a bowl and toss with the olive oil, making sure they're all lightly coated. Put the potatoes in one layer on a non-stick baking tray (or a baking tray covered with non-stick parchment or material) and bake for about 25 minutes, or until they're crisp and golden. I find there's no need to turn them during the cooking. Serve at once.

variation

low-fat lemony roast potatoes

Make these as described above, but mix the olive oil with the grated rind and juice of ½ a lemon before tossing with the potatoes.

fat-free garlicky roast potatoes

These potatoes are tender, golden and delectably garlicky. The vegetable stock adds flavour to this recipe – a stock cube or powder dissolved in hot water is fine.

serves 4

Preheat the oven to 230°C/450°F/gas mark 8.

Put the onion, garlic and vegetable stock into a shallow casserole dish large enough to hold the potatoes in one layer. Place the potatoes on top of the onion slices. Bake for 45–60 minutes until the potatoes are golden and there is no stock left, turning the potatoes over after about 30 minutes. Serve at once.

1 onion, sliced
6 large garlic cloves, roughly chopped
180ml/6fl oz/scant ¾ cup vegetable stock
500g/1lb 2oz small–medium potatoes, peeled and halved

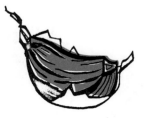

roast butternut squash with ginger

Roasting is a good way to cook butternut squash because it allows the full sweet flavour to come through undiluted by water. In this recipe the flavour is complemented by ginger, garlic and cumin. Yogurt and Fresh Herb Dressing (page 41) is excellent with it.

serves 4

1 butternut squash
2 garlic cloves, crushed
1tsp grated fresh ginger
1tsp ground cumin
salt and freshly ground
black pepper

Preheat the oven to 200°C/400°F/gas mark 6.

Cut the butternut squash, with its peel still on, into 5cm/2 in chunks, discarding the seeds. Put the crushed garlic, ginger and cumin into a bowl and mix to a paste. Rub the pieces of butternut squash into the paste so that the cut surfaces are all lightly coated. Season each piece with salt and freshly ground black pepper. Put the pieces in a single layer, skin-side down, on a shallow casserole dish and bake, uncovered, for about 40 minutes, until they feel very tender when pierced with a knife.

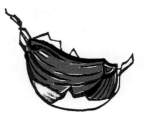

baked sweet potatoes with chive yogurt

Sweet potatoes with pinky-golden flesh are best for this dish. If you can't see this easily, make a small scratch on the skin to see the colour underneath. In this recipe, the chive yogurt contrasts well with the sweetness of the flesh.

serves 2

Preheat the oven to 200°C/400°F/gas mark 6.

Cut the sweet potatoes into chunky pieces, or leave them whole if you prefer and just prick the skins with a fork. Put the pieces in a single layer, skin-side down, on a shallow casserole dish and bake, uncovered, for about 30 minutes, until they are tender. The chunks will obviously cook more quickly than whole potatoes.

Meanwhile, mix the yogurt with the chives, and season with salt and freshly ground black pepper. To serve, break whole potatoes open and pour some of the yogurt and chive sauce inside, or pour the sauce over the chunks.

2 sweet potatoes, scrubbed
150ml/5fl oz/⅔ cup low-fat plain yogurt
1tbsp chopped fresh chives
salt and freshly ground black pepper

lemony cabbage

The best cabbage for this is a crisp green one like January King or the sweet and tender Sweetheart.

serves 2

225g/8oz cabbage, shredded
rind and juice of ½ a lemon
freshly grated nutmeg
salt and freshly ground black pepper

Bring 1cm/½ in of water to the boil in a saucepan. Put in the cabbage, cover and boil for about 4 minutes, or until just tender when pierced with the point of a sharp knife. Drain, then add the lemon rind and juice, and season with grated nutmeg, salt and freshly ground black pepper.

variations

cabbage with garlic

Boil shredded cabbage as described above. Drain the cabbage, return to the pan and add 1 crushed garlic clove. Stir the cabbage over the heat for a few seconds to cook the garlic. Season with salt and freshly ground black pepper and serve.

cabbage with nori

Cook and drain the cabbage, then sprinkle with nori powder before serving. You can buy this at large supermarkets and Oriental shops – it's nutritious as well as tasty.

baked beetroot with horseradish sauce

Prepared horseradish is available in several forms; I find the plain grated horseradish, in a jar, fine for this recipe.

serves 2

Preheat the oven to 200°C/400°F/gas mark 6.

Wrap each beetroot (beet) in a piece of foil, place on a baking tray and bake, uncovered, for about 1¼ hours, until the beetroots (beets) are tender.

To make the sauce, mix the yogurt with the horseradish and season with salt and freshly ground black pepper. Either unwrap the beetroots (beets) before serving, or serve them in their foil packages accompanied by the sauce: break open the packages and the beetroots (beets) and pour some of the horseradish sauce on top.

2 beetroots (beets), scrubbed
150ml/5fl oz/⅔ cup low-fat plain yogurt
1tsp grated horseradish
salt and freshly ground black pepper

carrots with lime and coriander

Carrots are versatile and can be enhanced by a variety of different flavourings. Cook them whole if they are very small, or in circles, batons or matchsticks if they're larger. Here the sharpness of the lime contrasts well with the natural sweetness of the carrots and the coriander (cilantro) emphasises the Oriental theme.

serves 2

250g/9oz carrots
grated rind and juice of
1 lime
1tbsp chopped fresh
coriander (cilantro)
salt and freshly ground
black pepper

Slice the carrots, or leave whole if small. Cover them in boiling water and cook until tender when pierced with a sharp knife. Drain and add the lime rind and juice, fresh coriander (cilantro) and some salt and freshly ground black pepper; toss the carrots gently, then serve.

carrots with caraway seeds

Caraway seed – also fennel and aniseed – enhance the sweet flavour of carrots. Add half a teaspoon to drained freshly-boiled carrots.

carrots with thyme

Thyme survives the drying process well, so either fresh or dried goes well with carrots. Add a teaspoonful of chopped fresh, or half a teaspoon of dried, after draining the carrots.

carrots with lemon and parsley

Toss drained carrots in the juice of half a lemon and 1 tablespoonful of chopped fresh parsley.

roasted mediterranean vegetables

These quantities are enough for a main course for two people or a first course or accompaniment for four.

serves 2–4

Preheat the oven to 230°C/450°F/gas mark 8.

Remove the stem from the aubergine (eggplant), cut the aubergine (eggplant) into chunks about 2.5 x 5cm/1 x 2 in and place in a large bowl. Add the oil and toss until coated all over. Place the aubergine (eggplant) chunks in a roasting pan. Cut the peppers into chunky strips, discarding the seeds and stems. Add the pepper strips to the roasting pan. (The pepper doesn't need any oil.) Place the pan near the top of the oven and roast for 20 minutes.

Turn the vegetables and add the artichoke hearts. Cook for a further 10 minutes, or until all the vegetables are tender and lightly browned. Season with salt and freshly ground black pepper and sprinkle with a little balsamic vinegar. Tear the basil, sprinkle over the vegetables and serve.

1 aubergine (eggplant)
1tsp olive oil
2 sweet red peppers
2 sweet golden peppers
400g/14oz can artichoke hearts, drained and halved
salt and freshly ground black pepper
balsamic vinegar
2–3 sprigs of basil

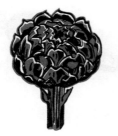

spicy parsnips and carrots

This is a nice way to add interest to root vegetables and works well with swede, as well as with parsnips and carrots.

serves 4

1 onion, finely chopped
225g/8oz carrots, cut into 5mm/¼ in dice
225g/8oz parsnips, peeled and cut into 5mm/¼ in dice
1tbsp curry powder
400ml/14fl oz/1¾ cups vegetable stock or water
salt and freshly ground black pepper
1–2tbsp chopped fresh parsley or coriander (cilantro), to serve

Put the onion into a non-stick pan, cover and cook gently for about 7 minutes, until the onion is tender and lightly browned, stirring from time to time. Add the carrot and parsnip. Stir, then turn down the heat, cover and leave to cook gently for a further 5 minutes, until the vegetables are getting tender, stirring often to prevent sticking. Stir in the curry powder and cook for a few seconds until it smells aromatic, then add 300ml/10fl oz/1¼ cups of the stock or water. Bring to the boil, then reduce the heat, cover and leave to boil gently for about 15 minutes, stirring occasionally, until the vegetables are very tender and most of the liquid has been absorbed. Add the rest of the stock or water during this time if necessary to keep the mixture moist while it cooks. Season with salt and freshly ground black pepper. Sprinkle with the fresh herbs before serving.

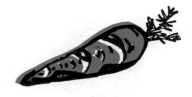

courgettes with mint

The refreshing flavour of mint really enlivens courgettes (zucchini).

serves 2

Bring 1cm/½ in of water to the boil in a saucepan.
Put in the courgettes (zucchini), cover and boil for 2–4
minutes, or until they are cooked to your taste – completely
tender or a bit on the crunchy side. Drain, then gently toss
the courgettes (zucchini) with the mint and some salt and
freshly ground black pepper.

225g/8oz courgettes
(zucchini), cut into rings,
batons or matchsticks
1–2tbsp chopped fresh mint
salt and freshly ground
black pepper

broccoli with cherry tomatoes

Broccoli in a rich tomato sauce is an Italian classic; here is a fresh, modern version, in which broccoli is half-boiled, half-steamed, then mixed with cherry tomatoes which are allowed to cook slightly in the heat of the pan. For a very pretty dish, use a mixture of red and yellow cherry tomatoes.

serves 4

500g/1lb 2oz broccoli
250g/9oz cherry tomatoes, halved
salt and freshly ground black pepper
6 large basil leaves, torn

Bring 1cm/½ in of water to the boil in a saucepan. Meanwhile, cut the broccoli into small florets, halving any larger ones. Cut the skin and stem ends off the stalks, then cut the inner stalks into matchsticks. Add the broccoli florets and matchsticks to the water when it boils, cover and boil for 3–4 minutes, or until the broccoli is cooked to your taste. The timing will depend on how tender it is, how big the pieces are, and how tender you like it. Drain the broccoli, return it to the hot pan and add the cherry tomatoes. Put the pan back on the heat, covered, for 30–60 seconds, until it starts to sizzle, then remove from the heat and leave to stand for 3–4 minutes, for the cherry tomatoes to cook. Season with salt and freshly ground black pepper, add the fresh basil and serve.

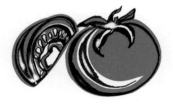

baked onions

Onions are wonderful when baked. They need no fat or other high calorie ingredients to enhance them.

Preheat the oven to 200°C/400°F/gas mark 6.

Put the onions into a baking tray and bake, uncovered, for about 45 minutes, until they are tender. Meanwhile, mix the yogurt with the chives, and season with salt and freshly ground black pepper. To serve, break the onions open and pour some of the yogurt and chive sauce inside; serve the rest of the sauce separately.

2 onions, unpeeled
150ml/5fl oz/⅔ cup low-fat plain yogurt
1tbsp chopped fresh chives
salt and freshly ground black pepper

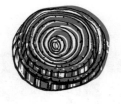

cabbage with butternut squash and sage

Cabbage and apple is a classic combination. In this recipe, butternut squash stands in admirably for the apple, its sweet softness contrasting pleasantly with crunchy cabbage. Some sage adds the final touch.

serves 2

225g/8oz cabbage, shredded
125g/4oz skinned butternut squash cut into 5mm/¼ in dice
8–12 fresh sage leaves, chopped
salt and freshly ground black pepper

Bring 1cm/½ in of water to the boil in a saucepan. Add the cabbage and squash, cover and boil for about 6 minutes, or until both squash and cabbage are tender. Drain, then stir in the sage and salt and freshly ground black pepper.

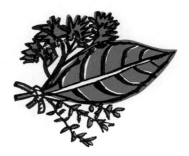

brussels sprouts with ginger

I'm sure the reasons why some people dislike Brussels sprouts are firstly that they're often overcooked and soggy, and secondly they have a natural sharp, slightly bitter flavour. Try cooking them this way – cut completely in half, which reduces the chance of overcooking them because it's easier to see when they're done, and tossed in grated fresh ginger, which has a naturally warm, sweet flavour.

serves 2

Bring 1cm/½ in of water to the boil in a saucepan. Add the Brussels sprouts, cover and boil for about 4 minutes, or until they are just tender when pierced with a skewer or the point of a sharp knife. Drain and put the sprouts back in the saucepan with the ginger and some salt and freshly ground black pepper. Toss gently over a moderate heat for a few seconds, to very lightly cook the ginger. The sprouts are best served immediately, though I think they're also very nice cold.

225g/8oz Brussels sprouts, halved
1–2tsps grated fresh ginger
salt and freshly ground black pepper

peas with lettuce and mint

Cooking frozen peas with a few lettuce leaves, some mint and spring (green) onions really brings out their flavour and makes them taste very much like fresh peas. (If you can get fresh peas, this is also a superb way to cook them.)

serves 2

225g/8oz/2 cups frozen or shelled peas
4 large lettuce leaves
4 spring (green) onions, chopped
4 large sprigs of fresh mint
salt and freshly ground black pepper

If you're using frozen peas straight from the freezer, put them into a sieve and pour boiling water on them to speed up the thawing process. Put the lettuce leaves into the base of a saucepan, then add the spring (green) onions, mint, peas and a sprinkling of salt and freshly ground black pepper. Cook over a gentle heat until the juices start to run and come to the boil; then cover and cook very gently for 4–5 minutes, or until the peas are heated through and tender.

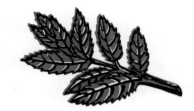

cauliflower with turmeric and cumin

I defy anyone to miss the fat or oil in this recipe. Cooked in this way, the cauliflower becomes golden, tender and lightly spiced. Turmeric has been shown to have properties which can help to protect from cancer, as well as giving the cauliflower an attractive colour and flavour.

serves 2

Put the onion into a non-stick saucepan and cook, without any additional fat or liquid, for 8–10 minutes, until it is tender and flecked with brown, stirring often to prevent sticking. Add the garlic, turmeric and cumin to the pan and stir over the heat for a further few seconds, until they smell aromatic. Then add the cauliflower, stock or water and some salt and freshly ground black pepper. Bring to the boil, cover, reduce the heat and leave to cook gently for about 8 minutes, or until the cauliflower is just tender and almost all the liquid has disappeared. Stir in the lemon juice, check the seasoning and serve.

1 onion, sliced
2 garlic cloves, crushed
¼ tsp turmeric powder
½ tsp cumin seeds
½ cauliflower, cut into small florets
100ml/3½ fl oz/scant ½ cup vegetable stock or water
salt and freshly ground black pepper
1tbsp freshly-squeezed lemon juice

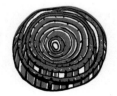

asparagus with golden pepper sauce

The sauce can be made well in advance and reheated just before serving. This has to be done carefully, however, as the yogurt in the sauce will separate if it gets anywhere near boiling. It's easier to make the sauce without the yogurt, reheat it and add the yogurt just before serving.

serves 2

225g/8oz asparagus
1 quantity Golden Pepper Sauce, page 134
salt and freshly ground black pepper

Break off the woody ends of the asparagus stems – if you bend them until they snap, they will naturally break where the stem gets really tough. Then, if you wish, use a potato peeler to peel a little way up the stem all the way round to remove the less tender part of the stem. Cook the asparagus by standing it up in a pan of boiling water, so that just the bottom part of the stems are in the water, or lay it flat in a large saucepan or frying pan so that the stems are completely submerged. Cook it for a few minutes, until it's tender to your liking, then drain it.

While the asparagus is cooking, gently reheat the golden pepper sauce. Put the asparagus on a plate, season with salt and freshly ground black pepper and serve with the sauce.

fat-free ratatouille

This ratatouille is moist, full of flavour and every bit as good as one made with lashings of oil.

serves 4

Put the onion into a non-stick saucepan and cook, without any additional fat or liquid, for 6–7 minutes, until it is flecked with brown, stirring often to prevent sticking. While the onion is cooking, peel the peppers using a swivel-bladed potato peeler to remove as much of the shiny skin as you can. Then deseed them and cut into slices. Add to the onion, along with the garlic, courgettes (zucchini) and aubergine (eggplant). Stir-fry for a minute or two and then add the chopped tomatoes in juice and a seasoning of salt and freshly ground black pepper. Bring to the boil, reduce the heat, cover and leave to cook gently for 25–30 minutes, until all the vegetables are tender. Sprinkle with chopped parsley and serve.

1 onion, sliced
2 sweet peppers, red, golden or a mixture
2 garlic cloves, crushed
2 courgettes (zucchini), sliced
1 aubergine (eggplant), cut into 5mm/¼ in dice
425g/15oz can chopped tomatoes in juice
salt and freshly ground black pepper
chopped fresh parsley, to serve

variation

spicy fat-free ratatouille

Ratatouille is also delicious with a flavouring of cumin and coriander. Follow the recipe above, adding 1 teaspoon of whole or ground cumin and 1 teaspoon of ground coriander to the onions just before adding the garlic. Stir for a few seconds over the heat until they smell aromatic, then add the garlic and other ingredients.

easy fennel niçoise

Tender, aniseed-flavoured fennel in a tomato sauce is delicious either hot or cold.

serves 2

350g/12oz fennel
1 quantity of Tomato Sauce,
page 133
grated rind and juice of
½ a lemon
salt and freshly ground
black pepper

Trim any green leafy bits from the fennel and set aside. Peel the outer layer of the fennel using a swivel-bladed potato peeler or sharp knife – this will get rid of any toughness. Slice the fennel.

Bring 1cm/½ in of water to the boil in a saucepan. Add the fennel, cover and boil gently for 8–10 minutes, or until the fennel is tender when pierced with a skewer or the point of a sharp knife. Drain the fennel (the water makes good stock).

Heat the tomato sauce in a pan, add the cooked fennel, lemon juice and rind and some salt and freshly ground black pepper. Cook over a gentle heat for 5–10 minutes, to allow the flavours to blend. Alternatively, you can mix together the fennel, sauce and lemon juice, cover and leave overnight. Next day, reheat gently or serve cold. In any case, snip any of the reserved leafy bits over the top of the dish before serving.

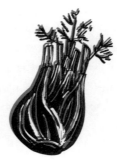

carrot and ginger mash

You can make this with carrots alone, or use a mixture of half carrots, half potatoes or other root vegetables – parsnips, turnips or swedes – for variations of flavour and texture. Both vegetables can cook together as long as they are cut into similar-sized pieces.

serves 4

Cover the carrots in boiling water and cook until they are very tender when pierced with a sharp knife. Drain, reserving the cooking water. Mash the carrots with the ginger, either with a potato masher or in a food processor or blender, adding a little of the cooking water to produce a soft consistency. Season with salt and freshly ground black pepper. If you're including potatoes in the mixture, it's best to mash them by hand rather than in a food processor which results in rather a gluey consistency.

500g/1lb 2oz carrots
1tsp grated fresh ginger
salt and freshly ground
black pepper

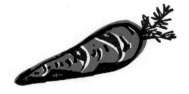

When I started thinking about low-fat cooking, I thought that sauces would be a problem. Obviously very rich sauces such as Hollandaise or Béarnaise are out and one accepts that, although both Golden Pepper Sauce (page 134) and Butternut Squash and Garlic Sauce (page 135) do go some way to filling that gap. But how to make a decent béchamel sauce without starting off with the traditional roux of butter and flour?

I found that by using soya milk it is possible to make a surprisingly creamy-tasting béchamel which can be flavoured with bay, parsley, onion, carrot and nutmeg. As far as the thickening is concerned, as I explained in the introduction, I haven't used wheat flour in this book but fine brown rice flour makes an excellent replacement. Of course there's no reason why you couldn't use wholewheat flour instead if you can eat it, though in fact I think that brown rice flour gives a better result.

Also included in this section is an onion gravy-type sauce, a dal sauce, tomato sauce and a zingy fresh tomato and ginger chutney.

béchamel sauce

This low-fat version of a classic sauce uses soya milk to give a particularly creamy result. Soya milk only has a little more fat than skimmed milk and is a very good milk replacement if you can't eat dairy products.

makes 300ml/ 10fl oz/1¼ cups

2tbsp brown rice flour
300ml/10fl oz/1¼ cups soya
or skimmed milk
1 bay leaf
sprig of parsley
small piece of onion and
carrot
salt and freshly ground
black pepper
grated nutmeg

Put the flour into medium-sized saucepan and mix to a paste with some of the milk. Gradually add the rest of the milk to produce a smooth consistency. Add the bay leaf, parsley, onion and carrot. Put the pan over a moderate heat and stir until thickened, then let it simmer very gently for 10 minutes to cook the flour. Remove the bay leaf, parsley, onion and carrot before serving, scraping as much of the sauce as you can from them back into the pan. Season with salt, freshly ground black pepper and nutmeg.

variations

onion sauce

Add one finely chopped onion after you've added the milk.

parsley sauce

For this fresh-tasting variation, add 1–2 tablespoons of finely chopped fresh parsley to the finished sauce.

leek sauce

Add 100g/3½ oz/ ⅔ cup finely sliced leek after you've added the milk.

tomato sauce

Tomato sauce is particularly useful in many recipes, and very easy to make.

serves 4

Put the onion into a non-stick pan, cover and cook gently for about 7 minutes, until the onion is tender and lightly browned, stirring from time to time. Add the garlic and cook for a few seconds. Add the tomatoes, chopping them up a bit in the pan with the spoon. Bring to the boil and leave to boil gently, uncovered, for 10–15 minutes, until the mixture is thick. Season with salt and freshly ground black pepper.

1 onion, chopped
1 large garlic clove, chopped
425g/15oz can tomatoes in juice
salt and freshly ground black pepper

variation

tomato and ginger sauce

For this lively variation, add 1–2 teaspoons finely chopped fresh ginger with the garlic.

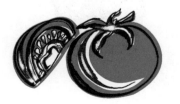

golden pepper sauce

This sauce seems much richer than it is simply because it looks a bit like buttery Hollandaise or Béarnaise sauce. It doesn't taste the same, although it has a creamy consistency and a sharp sweetness that results from the combination of sweet peppers, yogurt and mustard. The sauce enhances many delicate vegetable mixtures – try it with asparagus or with slim branches of cooked broccoli.

serves 4

1 large sweet golden pepper, deseeded and roughly chopped
1 garlic clove, chopped
2tbsp low-fat plain yogurt
½ tsp Dijon mustard
salt and freshly ground black pepper

Put the sweet pepper and garlic into a small saucepan, add about 1cm/¼ in of water, bring to the boil, cover and cook gently for 10–15 minutes, until the pepper is very tender. Drain, then put the chunks of pepper and garlic into a food processor or blender with the yogurt, mustard and some salt and freshly ground black pepper and whiz to a smooth purée. Taste and add more seasoning if necessary.

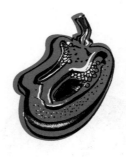

butternut squash and garlic sauce

This lovely creamy sauce is good for enlivening canned beans or freshly cooked vegetables.

serves 4

Preheat the oven to 200°C/400°F/gas mark 6.

Remove the seeds from the squash half and tuck the whole garlic cloves into the cavities. Put the halves cut-side down onto a baking tray and bake for 45–60 minutes, or until the butternut squash is tender when pierced with a knife or skewer. Cool, then scoop the flesh away from the skin using a spoon and discard the skin (but keep the garlic). All this can be done well in advance if convenient.

Put the butternut squash and garlic into a food processor or blender with the soya milk and some salt and freshly ground black pepper and whiz to a smooth, creamy sauce. Heat gently, without boiling.

½ butternut squash
6 garlic cloves
300ml/10fl oz/1¼ cups soya milk
salt and freshly ground black pepper

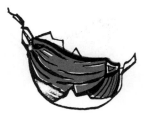

curry sauce

This sauce may have a lot of ingredients but it is quick and easy to make and an excellent way of jazzing up rather plain vegetables such as cauliflower. For a quick and healthy main course, try stirring cooked chick peas (garbanzo beans), butter or lima beans into it, then sprinkling with chopped fresh coriander (cilantro).

serves 4

1 onion, finely chopped
1 large garlic clove, finely chopped
1tsp grated fresh ginger
2½ tsp ground coriander
2½ tsp ground cumin
½ tsp curry powder
½ tsp turmeric
½ tsp white mustard seed
1 bay leaf
225g/8oz can tomatoes in juice
400ml/14fl oz/1¾ cups water
1tsp garam masala
salt and freshly ground black pepper

Put the onion into a non-stick pan, cover and cook gently for about 7 minutes, until the onion is tender and lightly browned, stirring from time to time. Add the garlic, fresh ginger and all the spices, except the garam masala, stirring over the heat for a few seconds until they smell aromatic. Add the tomatoes, chopping them up a bit in the pan with the spoon, and the water. Bring to the boil and leave to boil gently, uncovered, for 10–15 minutes, until the mixture is thickened a bit and no longer looks watery. Stir in the garam masala and season with salt and freshly ground black pepper.

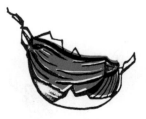

dal sauce

This sauce can turn a plate of ordinary steamed vegetables into a spicy and delicious low-fat main course – and it's very easy to make.

serves 3–4

Put the lentils into a saucepan with the onion, garlic, bay leaf, turmeric, ginger and water. Bring to the boil, then turn down the heat and leave to boil gently, uncovered, for 30–40 minutes, or until the lentils are very soft and the mixture is quite thick. There will be some froth on the water at first but don't worry about this; just stir the mixture and it will disappear as the lentils cook. Stir often towards the end of the cooking time to prevent sticking. When the lentils are thick and soft, stir in the cumin and coriander and season with salt and freshly ground black pepper.

200g/7oz/1 cup split red lentils
1 onion, chopped
1 large garlic clove, sliced
1 bay leaf
½ tsp ground turmeric
2 thin slices of fresh ginger
1 litre/35fl oz/4½ cups water
1tsp ground cumin
2tsp ground coriander
salt and freshly ground black pepper

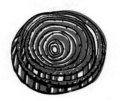

brown onion sauce

The important thing with this sauce is to make sure the onion is well browned.

serves 4

1 onion, chopped
1tbsp brown rice flour
300ml/10fl oz/1¼ cups vegetable stock
1 bay leaf
salt and freshly ground black pepper

Put the onion into a non-stick pan, cover and cook gently for about 7 minutes, until the onion is tender and well browned, stirring from time to time. Add the rice flour, stir over the heat for a minute, then stand well back and pour in the stock. Stir well until smooth, add the bay leaf and leave to simmer gently for 5–10 minutes. Add more stock if necessary to get the consistency you like. Season with salt and freshly ground black pepper.

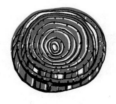

fresh tomato and ginger chutney

Quick to make and delicious with spicy dishes.

Mix all the ingredients together, seasoning with salt and freshly ground black pepper.

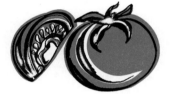

serves 4

225g/8oz tomatoes, sliced
or chopped
small piece of fresh ginger,
finely chopped
1tbsp freshly-squeezed
lemon juice
1 small onion or spring
(green) onion, sliced
3tbsp chopped fresh
coriander (cilantro)
salt and freshly ground
black pepper

desserts

As I explained in the general introduction, when deciding how strict to be in my interpretation of low sugar, I decided to take the 'pure' line: no fruit or artificial sweeteners. This is the advice given by many nutritional therapists, but there are few recipes which meet the criterion. (If your diet allows fruit and/or artificial sweeteners there is much more scope and plenty of recipes in other books.)

In this book I wanted to create some recipes for desserts which were not too different from normal, even though fruit, sugar and sweeteners were not allowed. If you are used to eating sugar, you will probably not find them sweet enough. However, once you have stopped eating sugar for a while, you will find, as I did when writing this book, that your appreciation of sweet things changes completely. Even vegetables such as carrots start to taste really sweet and certain ingredients such as carob powder, chestnut purée and butternut squash can be used very satisfactorily for sweetening. But, having said that, please don't expect the puddings in this section to taste anything like as sweet as normal ones.

Individual heatproof ramekin dishes (custard cups) are needed for the soufflés in this section and are also useful for serving cold desserts.

chestnut and carob soufflés

Serve these chocolatey little soufflés with Skimmed Milk Topping (page 154), or Vanilla Mousse (page 143).

serves 2

¼ x 425g/15oz can unsweetened chestnut purée
1tsp carob powder
2tsp real vanilla extract
1 egg white
2tbsp water

Preheat the oven to 200°C/400°F/gas mark 6 and position a baking tray towards the top.

Put the chestnut purée into a bowl and mash with a fork until it is lump-free. Add the carob powder, vanilla extract and water and beat again until completely smooth. Whisk the egg white until stiff peaks form. Stir a small tablespoonful of this into the chestnut mixture to loosen it. Add the chestnut mixture to the rest of the egg white. Very gently fold the two mixtures together using a metal spoon. Divide the mixture between two small ramekins (custard cups) and place these on the baking tray. Bake in the oven for 15–20 minutes until the soufflés have risen and are just firm in the centre. Serve at once.

vanilla mousse

The egg white is uncooked in this recipe; an organic free range egg from a reliable source should be fine but it's always wise to be on the safe side and not to eat it if you're in one of the vulnerable groups: lowered immunity, pregnant, elderly or very young.

serves 2

Put the yogurt into a bowl and stir in the vanilla extract. Whisk the egg white until it stands in stiff peaks. Stir a small tablespoonful of egg white into the yogurt to loosen it. Add the yogurt mixture to the rest of the egg white and fold them together. Divide between two glasses, chill and serve with the raspberry sauce. The mousse can also be chilled and used as a topping.

150ml/5fl oz/ ⅔ cup very low-fat plain yogurt
2tsp real vanilla extract
1 egg white
1 quantity Raspberry Sauce, page 152

variation

raspberry and vanilla layer

Spoon a little of the vanilla mixture into two glasses, alternating with spoonfuls of raspberry sauce, to create a stripy knickerbocker glory effect. Chill and serve.

little rice soufflés with raspberry sauce

Break open the crunchy top of this soufflé, pour in a little of the sauce, eat and enjoy.

serves 2

25g/1oz/3tbsp flaked brown rice
300ml/10fl oz/1¼ cups soya milk
2tsps real vanilla extract
1 egg white
1 quantity Raspberry Sauce, page 152

Preheat the oven to 200°C/400°F/gas mark 6.

Put the flaked rice into a saucepan with the milk. Bring to the boil over a moderate heat, stirring. Reduce the heat and leave the rice to cook gently, uncovered, for 5 minutes, until thick and creamy. Stir in the vanilla extract.

Whisk the egg white until it stands in stiff peaks. Stir a small tablespoonful of egg white into the rice mixture to loosen it. Add the rice mixture to the rest of the egg white and fold them together. Transfer the mixture to two ramekins (custard cups). Bake for 15–20 minutes until puffed up and set. Serve with the raspberry sauce.

little lemon soufflés

These little soufflés are good on their own, or with one of the fruit sauces (page 152).

(page 152)

serves 2

Preheat the oven to 200°C/400°F/gas mark 6.

Remove the seeds from the squash half, then put it cut-side down on to a baking tray and bake for 45–60 minutes, or until it's tender. Cool, then scoop the flesh away from the skin using a spoon and discard the skin. All this can be done well in advance if convenient.

Mash the butternut squash with a fork or purée it in a food processor or blender. Add the grated lemon rind. Whisk the egg white until it stands in stiff peaks. Stir a small tablespoonful of egg white into the butternut purée to loosen it. Add the butternut purée to the rest of the egg white and fold them together. Transfer the mixture to two ramekins (custard cups). Bake in the oven for 15–20 minutes until puffed up and set.

½ butternut squash
finely grated rind of ½ a well-scrubbed organic lemon
1 egg white

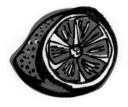

ground rice pudding with blackcurrant sauce

Use brown rice flour, from health food stores, for this soothing pudding.

serves 1–2

2tbsp brown rice flour
300ml/10fl oz/1¼ cups soya milk
1tsp real vanilla extract, optional
1 quantity Blackcurrant Sauce, page 152

Put the rice flour into a saucepan and gradually blend with the milk. Heat gently, stirring, until the mixture thickens. Leave to simmer over a very gentle heat for 5–10 minutes, to cook the rice flour. Add the vanilla extract if you're using this, and serve with the blackcurrant sauce.

butternut squash crumble

You can buy flaked brown rice at good health food stores along with other flaked grains such as millet, which can also be used in this recipe. Serve on its own or with Custard (page 155).

serves 2

Preheat the oven to 200°C/400°F/gas mark 6.

Remove the seeds from the squash half, then put it cut-side down onto a baking tray and bake for 45–60 minutes, or until it's tender. Cool, then scoop the flesh away from the skin using a spoon and discard the skin. All this can be done well in advance if convenient.

Mash the butternut squash with a fork or cut it into small chunks. Either way, mix it with the grated lemon rind and put it into a shallow casserole dish. Scatter the flaked rice evenly on top and bake in the preheated oven for about 20 minutes, or until the flaked rice is lightly browned.

½ butternut squash
grated rind of ½ a lemon
3tbsp flaked brown rice

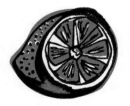

flaked rice pudding

This is good either hot or cold, on its own or accompanied by a fruit sauce (page 152).

serves 1

25g/1oz/3tbsp flaked brown rice
300ml/10fl oz/1¼ cups soya milk
1tsp real vanilla extract

Put the flaked rice into a saucepan with the milk. Bring to the boil over a moderate heat, stirring. Reduce the heat and leave the rice to cook gently, uncovered, for 5 minutes, until thick and creamy. Stir in the vanilla extract and serve.

variations

cinnamon rice

Omit the vanilla extract and instead sprinkle ¼ teaspoon ground cinnamon over the rice before serving.

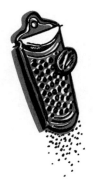

nutmeg rice

Omit the vanilla extract and grate some nutmeg over the top before serving.

lemon rice

Add the finely grated rind of half a small lemon to the flaked rice and milk; cook as described above but omit the vanilla extract. Some Raspberry Sauce (page 156) is particularly delicious with this version.

flaked millet pudding

Make exactly as above using flaked millet instead of flaked brown rice.

golden vanilla cream

Sweet and very creamy, this makes a wonderful low-sugar, low-fat dessert. It's worth getting good vanilla extract; you can buy Madagascar Bourbon vanilla extract at high class food shops and in the special selections at some large supermarkets.

serves 2

½ butternut squash
150ml/5fl oz/⅔ cup soya milk
1–2tsp vanilla extract
1 egg white, optional

Preheat the oven to 200°C/400°F/gas mark 6.

Remove the seeds from the squash half, then put it cut-side down onto a baking tray and bake for 45–60 minutes, or until it's tender. Cool, then scoop the flesh away from the skin using a spoon and discard the skin. All this can be done well in advance if convenient.

Put the butternut squash into a food processor or blender with the soya milk and whiz to a smooth, creamy sauce. Add vanilla extract to taste. Pour into individual glasses and chill; or, if you're using the egg white, whisk until standing in soft peaks, then fold this into the butternut mixture. Spoon into glasses and chill.

variation

golden vanilla sauce

This thinner version of the cream is a good custard substitute. Simply omit the egg white and gently heat the mixture after adding the vanilla extract, instead of chilling it.

red jelly

I really don't know what to say about this recipe except try it; don't let the ingredients put you off. If you're buying cooked beetroot (beet), make sure it's been prepared without vinegar. Vegetable substitutes for gelatine, such as gelozone, can be bought from health shops. The jelly is nice served with a dollop of plain yogurt, Vanilla Mousse (page 143) or the Skimmed Milk Topping (page 154).

serves 2

4 raspberry tea bags (or a mixture)
150ml/5fl oz/⅔ cup boiling water
½ tsp gelozone or vege-gel
1 small cooked beetroot (beet), finely chopped

Put the tea bags into a bowl, pour over the boiling water and leave for at least 30 minutes to infuse. Then squeeze out the tea bags to extract as much of the flavour as possible. Discard the tea bags. Divide the beetroot (beet) between two dessert glasses. Heat the fruity tea in a small saucepan, sprinkle over the gelozone or vege-gel and bring to the boil, stirring. Boil for 1 minute, then pour over the beetroot (beet) and leave to set.

soya yogurt

Although you can buy unsweetened soya yogurt, it's not easy to come by and you might prefer to make your own. This is very easy to do, using unsweetened soya milk and a starter of very low fat organic (milk) yogurt. Once you've made your first batch, you can use some of your own soya yogurt to start subsequent batches.

If you haven't got a yogurt maker, you can use a wide-neck thermos flask or create a warm place to incubate the yogurt. I use a large polystyrene box – or a cool box would do. I fill a hot water bottle with water in the normal way, place it in the bottom of the box and stand the 450g/16oz jars of yogurt-to-be, three or six at a time on another thick piece of polystyrene (an old blanket would do) on top of the hot water bottle. I then put a padding of tea towels around them and cover the box with the lid. After 8 hours, or overnight, there's a batch of perfectly set soya yogurt which keeps for 2–3 weeks in the refrigerator. One litre/35fl oz/4½ cups of soya milk is just the right quantity to fill three empty 450g/1lb honey or marmalade jars. Sterilise the jars and lids by putting them in the dishwasher or washing well and filling with boiling water before using them.

makes 1 litre/ 35fl oz/4½ cups

Heat the milk until it feels hot to your little finger but not so hot that you have to pull it out immediately. Put a teaspoonful of the yogurt into your three jars. Pour a little of the soya milk into each and quickly stir to distribute the yogurt, then top up with the rest of the milk. Put on the lids, and put the jars into the cosy nest you have created. Or of course pour the milk and yogurt mixture into a wide-mouthed vacuum flask or the jars of a yogurt maker. Leave for 8 hours, or until the yogurt has set.

1 litre/35fl oz/ 4½ cups unsweetened organic soya milk
3tsp soya or very low fat dairy yogurt

raspberry sauce

Fruit tea bags (check the packet to make sure they haven't any added sweetening – most haven't) can be used to make delicious sugar-free sauces. There are plenty of different flavourings to choose from. This sauce is made from raspberry tea bags and is excellent with creamy cereal puddings or poured over yogurt.

serves 4

4 raspberry tea bags
150ml/5fl oz/⅔ cup boiling water
1tsp potato flour (starch)

Put the tea bags into a bowl, pour over the boiling water and leave for at least 30 minutes to infuse. Squeeze out the tea bags to extract as much of the flavour as possible. Discard the tea bags. Put the arrowroot (potato starch) into a small saucepan, add a little of the tea and mix to a paste, then add the rest of the tea. Place over a gentle heat and stir until thickened. Use hot or cold.

variations

blackcurrant sauce

This is made as above using blackcurrant tea bags instead of raspberry.

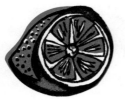

lemon and ginger sauce

Use lemon and ginger tea bags instead of the raspberry. Add the grated rind of ½ a lemon.

chestnut and carob sauce

Serve this sauce over low-fat plain yogurt or with Vanilla Mousse (page 143). The recipe only uses a quarter of a can of chestnut purée but the remainder will keep well for a couple of days in the refrigerator, or for 3–4 weeks in the freezer.

serves 4

Put the chestnut purée into a bowl and mash with a fork, or whiz in a food processor or blender until it is lump-free. Add the carob powder, vanilla extract and water and whiz or beat again until everything is completely blended and the sauce is smooth and glossy.

¼ x 425g/15oz can unsweetened chestnut purée
1tsp carob powder
2tsp real vanilla extract
150ml/5fl oz/ ⅔ cup water

skimmed milk topping

If you can take milk, this is a useful creamy-tasting yet practically fat-free topping. You do need an electric whisk to make it and it's essential to use skimmed milk powder (not granules and not a milk-substitute powder), which you may have to buy from a health food store.

serves 4–6

40g/1½ oz skimmed milk powder
150ml/5fl oz/⅔ cup ice-cold water
2tbsp freshly-squeezed lemon juice
½ tsp real vanilla extract

Put the skimmed milk powder and water into a bowl and beat with an electric whisk for 4–5 minutes, until the mixture is thick and forms stiff peaks. Add the lemon juice and vanilla extract and whisk again until the soft peaks form again. Use within a few hours.

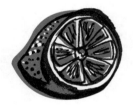

custard

Using polenta, which like cornflour (cornstarch) is made from maize, gives this recipe a certain comforting resemblance to custard, as does the golden colour.

serves 1–2

Put the polenta into a saucepan and gradually blend with the soya milk and vanilla extract. Heat gently, stirring, until the mixture thickens. Leave to simmer over a very gentle heat for 5–10 minutes, to cook the polenta.

2tsp fine instant polenta
150ml/5fl oz/⅔ cup soya milk
1tsp real vanilla extract

The challenges of making low-fat, low-sugar desserts which I described at the beginning of the last section apply, perhaps to an even greater degree, when it comes to making breads and cakes. This is therefore quite a short and select section which I hope will prove useful in providing a few treats if you're on a very restricted diet.

breads and cakes

soda bread

Easy to make and completely fat-free, soda bread can be made from wholewheat flour or mixtures of other flours such as oatmeal, cornmeal and rice flour.

makes 1 loaf

450g/1lb/3 cups plus 3tbsp plain (all-purpose) wholewheat flour

1tsp bicarbonate of soda (baking soda)

2tsp freshly-squeezed lemon juice

300–350ml/10–12fl oz/ 1¼–1½ cups soya milk

extra flour for coating

Preheat the oven to 200°C/400°F/gas mark 6.

Put the flour into a bowl and mix in the bicarbonate of soda (baking soda). Add the lemon juice and mix to a soft dough with the milk. The dough needs to be soft but able to hold its shape. Turn the dough out onto a floured board and knead very lightly into a circle. Place on a baking tray and cut a cross in the top of the loaf. Bake for about 30 minutes, until the loaf sounds hollow when you turn it upside down and rap it with your knuckles. Cool on a wire rack – or eat the bread while it's still warm. It's best eaten the same day but freezes well. Make sure it's completely cold before freezing.

carrot and rosemary flatbread

This is a moist flatbread with a cake-like texture. Eat it very fresh as an accompaniment to cooked casseroles, chillis and stews.

serves 4

Preheat the oven to 200°C/400°F/gas mark 6. Line a 20cm/8 in square baking pan with non-stick baking parchment.

Put the rice flour into a bowl with the bicarbonate of soda (baking soda), salt and two teaspoons of the rosemary and mix together. Whisk together the egg white, soya milk and lemon juice and add to the dry ingredients in the bowl along with the onion and carrot. Mix quickly to a batter, then pour into the prepared baking pan. Sprinkle the remaining rosemary on top and bake for 15–20 minutes, or until firm in the middle and golden brown on top. Serve hot or warm.

100g/3½ oz/⅔ cup brown rice flour
½ tsp bicarbonate of soda (baking soda)
½ tsp salt
3tsp chopped fresh rosemary
1 egg white
150ml/5fl oz/⅔ cup soya milk
1tsp freshly-squeezed lemon juice
1 small onion, chopped
100g/3½ oz/½ cup grated carrot

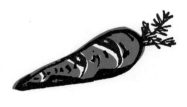

oatcakes

This is a slight adaptation of my favourite oatcake recipe which is in *Food Combining for Health*, by Doris Grant and Jean Joice. In this version I have omitted the level teaspoonful of unsalted butter, to make low-fat oatcakes which are crisp and delicious. They are wonderful with dips, or on their own, when you want something crunchy to eat.

makes 16

150g/5oz/1¼ cups medium oatmeal
½ tsp salt
125ml/4fl oz/½ cup boiling water
extra oatmeal for rolling out

Preheat the oven to 200°C/400°F/gas mark 6.

Put the oatmeal into a bowl with the salt and water. Mix, then leave for a minute or so for the oatmeal to swell. Turn the mixture out on a board sprinkled with oatmeal. Divide into two pieces. Roll each into a circle and cut into 8 pieces. Roll each of the 8 pieces to make them as thin as you can. If you roll them from edge to edge, rather than from the point to the edge, they will stay a good triangle shape. Put them onto a baking tray and bake for about 12 minutes until they are crisp and light golden. I sometimes turn them over once the top has set (after about 6–7 minutes) to do the other side, but this isn't essential. Cool on a wire rack and keep in an airtight container.

lemon muffins

Use paper muffin cases for these to prevent the muffins sticking to their baking pan.

makes 6

Preheat the oven to 200°C/400°F/gas mark 6. Stand the muffin cases on a baking tray or in the sections of a muffin pan.

Prepare the squash. Remove the seeds from the squash half, then put it cut-side down onto a baking tray and bake for 45–60 minutes, or until it's tender. Cool, then scoop the flesh away from the skin using a spoon and discard the skin. Mash the butternut squash with a fork and leave to cool. All this can be done well in advance if convenient.

Put the rice flour, bicarbonate of soda (baking soda) and grated lemon rind into a bowl and mix together. Whisk together the egg white, soya milk, lemon juice and vanilla extract and add to the dry ingredients in the bowl along with the butternut squash. Mix quickly to a smooth, thick consistency, then put large tablespoonfuls of the mixture into the paper cases. Bake in the preheated oven for 20–25 minutes, or until firm in the middle.

½ butternut squash
100g/3½ oz/ ⅔ cup brown rice flour
½ tsp bicarbonate of soda (baking soda)
grated rind of 1 lemon
1 egg white
150ml/5fl oz/ ⅔ cup soya milk
1tsp lemon juice
1tsp real vanilla extract

6 paper muffin cases

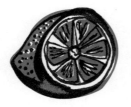

chestnut and carob truffles

Like the other chestnut recipes in this book, you only need a quarter of a can of chestnut purée to make these truffles. The remainder will keep well for a couple of days in the refrigerator, or for 3–4 weeks in the freezer.

makes 8
serves 4

¼ x 425g/15oz can unsweetened chestnut purée
1tsp carob powder
2tsp real vanilla extract
2tbsp water
a little extra carob powder to coat

Put the chestnut purée into a bowl and mash with a fork until it is lump-free. Add the carob powder, vanilla extract and water and mix to a paste. Form into small balls and coat in a little extra carob powder.

carob brownies

Butternut squash adds sweetness and moisture to these brownies. Prepare the butternut squash beforehand as described in the recipe for Lemon Muffins (page 161).

makes 16

Preheat the oven to 200°C/400°F/gas mark 6. Line a 20cm/8 in square baking pan with non-stick baking parchment.

Put the rice flour into a bowl with the carob powder, ginger, cinnamon and bicarbonate of soda (baking soda) and mix together. Whisk together the egg white, soya milk and lemon juice and add to the dry ingredients in the bowl along with the mashed butternut squash. Mix quickly to a smooth, thick consistency, then pour into the prepared baking pan. Bake for 15–20 minutes, or until firm in the middle. Cool in the pan, then cut into 16 squares and remove from the pan.

100g/3½ oz/ ⅔ cup brown rice flour
1tbsp carob powder
½ tsp ground ginger
¼ tsp ground cinnamon
½ tsp bicarbonate of soda (baking soda)
1 egg white
150ml/5fl oz/ ⅔ cup soya milk
1tsp freshly-squeezed lemon juice
200g/7 oz cooked butternut squash, page 161

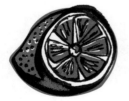

lemon cake
with blackcurrant filling

Keep this cake in the refrigerator and eat within a couple of days or so. Prepare the butternut squash beforehand as described in the recipe for Lemon Muffins (page 161).

makes one cake

100g/3½ oz/⅔ cup brown rice flour
½ tsp bicarbonate of soda (baking soda)
grated rind of 1 lemon
1 egg white
150ml/5fl oz/⅔ cup soya milk
1tsp freshly-squeezed lemon juice
1tsp real vanilla extract
200g/7oz cooked butternut squash, page 161

for the filling
4 blackcurrant tea bags
150ml/5fl oz/⅔ cup boiling water
1tbsp potato flour (starch)

Preheat the oven to 180°C/350°F/gas mark 4. Line the base of two 17cm/7 in sponge tins (cake pans) with non-stick baking parchment.

Put the rice flour, bicarbonate of soda (baking soda) and grated lemon rind into a bowl and mix together. Whisk together the egg white, soya milk, lemon juice and vanilla extract and add to the dry ingredients in the bowl along with the mashed butternut squash. Mix quickly to a smooth, thick consistency, then divide between the two prepared tins (pans). Bake for 10–15 minutes, or until firm in the middle. Cool for a few minutes in the tins (pans), then turn out onto a cooling rack and leave until completely cold.

Meanwhile, make the blackcurrant filling. Put the tea bags into a bowl, cover with the boiling water and leave to infuse for 30 minutes. Remove the tea bags, squeezing them in your hands to extract all the liquid. Put the potato flour (starch) into a small saucepan and blend to a paste with the blackcurrant liquid. Stir over the heat for a few minutes, until the mixture has thickened. Remove from the heat and cool.

Put one of the cakes upside down on a plate, spread the blackcurrant mixture evenly over and place the other cake on top.

carob cake with chestnut carob filling

Like the previous cake, Carob Cake is made with cooked butternut squash which needs to be prepared beforehand. The cake needs to be eaten within a couple of days and is best kept covered in the refrigerator.

makes one cake

Preheat the oven to 180°C/350°F/gas mark 4. Line the base of two 17.5cm/7 in sponge tins (cake pans) with non-stick baking parchment.

Put the rice flour, carob powder and bicarbonate of soda (baking soda) into a bowl and mix together. Whisk together the egg white, soya milk, lemon juice and vanilla extract and add to the dry ingredients in the bowl along with the mashed butternut squash. Mix quickly to a smooth, thick consistency, then divide between the two prepared tins (pans). Bake for 10–15 minutes, or until firm in the middle. Cool for a few minutes in the tins (pans), then turn out onto a cooling rack and leave until completely cold. Sandwich the cakes with the chestnut carob spread.

100g/3½ oz/ ⅔ cup brown rice flour
1tbsp carob powder
½ tsp bicarbonate of soda (baking soda)
1 egg white
150ml/5fl oz/ ⅔ cup soya milk
1tsp freshly-squeezed lemon juice
2tsp real vanilla extract
200g/7oz cooked butternut squash, page 161

for the filling
Chestnut Carob Spread, page 24

index

Cheap and Easy

ROSE ELLIOT

Regarded by many vegetarians as the cookery bible, *Cheap and Easy* — now completely revised and updated — is a collection of over 150 inspiring recipes that demonstrate that tasty and nutritious dishes, such as Nut Roast or Couscous with Spicy Bean Stew, can be accomplished both simply and economically. *Cheap and Easy* will be an invaluable addition to any bookshelf.

Internationally renowned as a vegetarian cookery writer, Rose Elliot's other books include *Low Fat, Low Sugar*, *Vegetarian Christmas* and *Vegan Feasts*.

The Bean Book

ROSE ELLIOT

This new edition of the vegetarian classic cookbook gives the low-down on beans and pulses of every flavour, colour and variety.

Beans are not only delicious – they are terrific sources of essential proteins and are the ultimate healthy food. With recipes such as West Indian Red Beans and Lentil Pie, even the non-vegetarian will be converted to the versatile pulse!

Internationally renowned as a vegetarian cookery writer, Rose Elliot's other books include *Low Fat, Low Sugar, Cheap and Easy* and *Vegan Feasts*.

Thorsons

Directions for life

www.thorsons.com

The latest mind, body and spirit news

Exclusive author interviews

Read extracts from the latest books

Join in mind-expanding discussions

Win great prizes every week

Thorsons catalogue & ordering service

www.thorsons.com